American Diet Revolution!

American Diet Revolution!

The Strength for Life® Guide to the Foods
We Must and Must Not Eat To Be Leaner
and Stronger in the 21st Century

Dr. Josef Arnould

NEW YORK

LONDON • NASHVILLE • MELBOURNE • VANCOUVER

American Diet Revolution!

The Strength for Life® Guide to the Foods We Must and Must Not Eat To Be Leaner and Stronger in the 21st Century

Published in New York, New York, by Morgan James Publishing. Morgan James is a trademark of Morgan James, LLC. www.MorganJamesPublishing.com

ISBN 9781642791082 paperback
ISBN 9781642791099 eBook
Library of Congress Control Number: 2018945522

Cover Design by:
Megan Dillon
megan@creativeninjadesigns.com

Interior Design by:
Chris Treccani
www.3dogcreative.net

Interior Illustrations by:
Alan Robinson

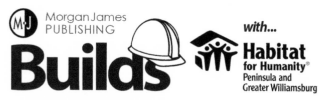

Morgan James is a proud partner of Habitat for Humanity Peninsula and Greater Williamsburg. Partners in building since 2006.

Get involved today! Visit
MorganJamesPublishing.com/giving-back

This work is dedicated to any person:

who seeks honest, up-to-date, nutritional information;

who yearns to eat as healthfully as possible;

who has tried many different diet plans to lose excessive body fat,

but has yet to attain long-term success;

who has ever been confused by conflicting dietary advice;

who believes the scientific method should be applied truthfully

to research in the fields of nutrition and weight loss;

who struggles with diabetes, dementia, or other diet-mediated diseases;

who is willing to try delicious new foods and delicious old foods;

who is concerned about how our food choices affect

our local communities, our nation, and our planet;

who refuses to be a passive acceptor of dietary misinformation;

who always embraces the challenge to be an active questioner of everything;

and, who is willing to revolt against all individuals and organizations that deceive us

about the qualities of the foods we must eat

to achieve the freedom of good health.

Table of Contents

Acknowledgments

For their inspiration and assistance in the composition and revisions of this work, I offer special thanks to:

- Tito Gambarini, painter, long-retired surgeon, and nonagenarian strength trainee, whose brilliantly colored and dynamic paintings dance upon the walls of the Strength for Life® Fitness Center and inspire all of us to live every day with humor and gusto;
- Alan Robinson, graphic artist extraordinaire, for creating visual representations of dietary and fitness reformation;
- Ella Boliver, for the illustration of Milo of Croton, five-time Olympic champion and mascot of the Strength for Life® Health & Fitness Center;
- Abby Arnould, my patient wife, who endures countless middle-of-the-night arousals as the churning of ideas propels me back to my desk;
- My fellow and sister trainees and staff members at Strength for Life® Health & Fitness Center, who share with me the incredible joy and excitement of exercising vigorously every day;
- Richard Muise, Steve Dinkelaker, Charlotte Vesel, Caitlin Arnould, and Lori Steiner, who have critiqued this work constructively; and

- In memoriam, Charlie Hatfield, whose witticisms made life a lot more fun and a little more puzzling for all of us who were fortunate to share time and the exhilaration of exercise with him over the past three decades.

For their professional guidance, editorial skills, and publishing expertise in elevating this work from a mere manuscript to a book worthy of publication, I am indebted deeply to:

- Aubrey Kosa, my frontline editor par excellence, for correcting my editorial transgressions and for breathing conversational life and clarity into the text;
- Tiffany Gibson, my Author Relations Manager, for navigating this work through the locks and dams of the publishing process;
- Jim Howard, Publisher at Morgan James Publishing, for transforming a simple typed manuscript into an exciting instrument of learning that appeals to your eyes and feels great in your hands;
- David Hancock, visionary founder of Morgan James Publishing, not only for accepting my manuscript, but for sharing his contagious enthusiasm for learning with real books in the 21st Century;
- Ruth Klein, my agent and marketing strategist, for taking me from the rocking chair of "Let's see what's going to happen," to the rocket of "Let's show the whole world what you really have to offer!"

Introduction

I wish this book could be simply a straightforward plan to achieve excellent health by eating nutritious and delicious foods. When I began this work, my only intentions were (1) to summarize the most credible nutritional research findings of the 21st Century and (2) to distill that information into easy-to-follow dietary guidelines for the patients and exercise trainees in the Strength for Life® clinic.

For two very compelling reasons, I found that limiting the scope of this book to my original modest intentions would be to tell only half of a very complex story. First, the fields of dietary advice and nutritional research are littered with so many conflicting bits of information from so many different sources that it is very difficult for most of us to judge which sources to believe and which to disregard. If we are to make informed dietary choices, we must understand the history of nutritional research, agricultural economics, and other factors that have shaped the major dietary movements in the United States—not just during the 21st Century, but for the last half of the 20th Century as well. Each of us must do a little personal investigating. We cannot trust any single "expert." Instead, you and I must read at least one or two books by honest nutritionists, researchers, scientific writers, or physicians of the 21st Century. Only by reading and thinking for ourselves do we become capable of judging which authorities can be trusted and which cannot.

The second—and even more important—reason I chose to exceed my original intentions is that the epidemics of obesity, diabetes, drug addiction, dementia, and other diet-related diseases continue to surge, not only in the US, but worldwide. To publish yet another politely written book of dietary advice would not be sufficiently motivational for enough people to take the radical actions necessary to reverse the upward trends of these preventable and prematurely disabling diseases. Improving your own personal diet is merely a first step. As members of highly interconnected local, national, and international communities, we are all affected adversely by these epidemics. We must face these enemies to our collective health freedom. The costs of being passive—of allowing preventable diseases to continue expanding—threaten to overwhelm the economy of the richest nation in human history. Even though these diseases have been recognized for decades, thus far, the tactics employed to overcome them have been much too feeble. Only a full-scale revolt against the foods many of us still eat—and what we think about the foods we eat—can bring about the profound changes in our health that must occur if we are to survive and thrive as individuals, as nations, and as a species. I contend that most of us will be motivated to advocate forcefully for society-wide dietary reforms when, and only when, we learn about the clandestine activities of prominent individuals and groups who have used dietary misinformation to profit immensely at great expense to our health during the last half of the 20th Century and beyond. My hypothesis is this: if I can stir up widespread outrage, greater numbers of us will choose to take meaningful action than if I were to only present a sensible dietary plan.

If I state that eating a bowl of oatmeal with banana slices or raisins and drinking a glass of orange juice for breakfast every day will cause you to gain unwanted body fat and/or prevent you from losing it, a significant percentage of readers will doubt the truthfulness of that statement and be unwilling to eliminate those foods from their diets. And if I state that you can enhance your health and decrease your body fat by eating whole eggs from pasture-raised chickens, homemade sauerkraut, and raw dandelion greens every day, an equally sizeable percentage of readers will doubt or ignore such advice. However, if I cite detailed, up-to-date research findings that support such assertions, those same skeptical readers will at least *consider* my dietary recommendations. Furthermore, if I cite evidence that certain well-respected economic and medical groups have conspired to keep us eating foods that have made us increasingly obese, an even greater number of readers will take notice and consider the dietary information presented by 21st Century nutritional research.

In the first half of this book, I summarize the history of dietary research and advice in the US in the last half of the 20th Century. Only by exploring that disturbing history can we begin to understand how and why corrupt dietary recommendations during that crucial period caused such devastating increases in obesity and its related diseases. Unfortunately, consciously or not, most Americans still follow those same recommendations.

Next, I contrast the deceptions of the 20th Century with works of several independent researchers and writers of the 21st Century who dare to document the deliberate deceptions of their predecessors. These new authors are not mere naysayers. They explain not only which foods we should no longer eat, but also the types of foods we must restore to our diets if we wish to be lean and healthy. Several of these authors offer extensive menus, recipes, and preparation techniques for beneficial foods to put back into our diets in pursuit of regaining the freedom of good health.

In the second half of this book, based upon my understanding of the most scientifically supported nutritional research of the 21st Century, I present my specific dietary recommendations. In addition, I propose personal action steps each of us can take to regain our health freedom from the conspiring economic groups who colonized us in the past with deceptive nutritional advice.

Have you ever tried an energy drink made only of wheat germ oil and blackstrap molasses? Beginning with a few books from my high school library in the early 1960s, I have been studying nutrition for over 50 years. I have taken more nutritional wrong turns than anyone you know. Obediently, I accepted dietary advice from the United States Department of Agriculture and other prestigious groups I assumed I could trust. I tried being a vegetarian, a vegan, eating egg whites and throwing away the yolks as part of a low-fat diet, making blueberry preserves with fructose, drinking skim milk and soy milk, eating lots of organic whole grains, etc. In short, like many of you during the last half of the 20th Century, I lived through and experienced first-hand a great deal of nutritional confusion.

Fortunately, since the beginning of the present millennium, a new wave of dedicated and independent nutritional researchers and writers has arisen. They have documented meticulously the fallacies, mistakes, and oftentimes the deliberate deceptions in the dietary advice put forth to us in the last half of the 20th Century by governmental agencies, by celebrated academics, and by what once were thought to be respectable and responsible medical and scientific organizations. These recent nutritional writers have demanded that the scientific method, rather than financial profits, be restored as the basis from which nutritional advice should be developed, verified, and disseminated. Not only have they exposed the errors and deceits of their predecessors, but, collectively, they have proposed sweeping changes in the types of foods we eat. In short, they have cleared the weeds of confusion from the field of nutrition and planted seeds for a revolution in the American diet.

As a practicing Doctor of Chiropractic for over 30 years, I have observed—as well as witnessed with both hands—that many patients add 20, 40, 60, or more pounds of fat to their bodies over the course of one or two decades. Not only do I feel the gradual accumulation of excess fat on their torsos and limbs, but I also often measure it objectively with bioimpedance analysis (BIA). An inordinately high percentage of these patients suffer from severe inflammatory symptoms—not only joint and muscular aches and pains, but also gastrointestinal problems, autoimmune diseases, depression, skin disorders, stomach cancer, and so on. When I counsel patients about their diets and recommend changes in their eating habits, I am amazed that so many remain confused about the dietary causes of weight gain. They still cling to the nutritional advice they heard over and over during the last half of the 20th Century. They say:

"It can't be my diet because I eat really healthy."

"I don't eat very much, but I still gain weight."

"I always watch what I eat, but it doesn't seem to make much difference."

"I don't understand why I keep getting fat. I always buy nonfat foods."

"My cholesterol keeps going up even though I try not to eat any foods that have cholesterol in them."

"My mother started to put on weight too when she reached my age."

To help patients and trainees with weight-gain problems, I recommend gradual, specific changes in their personal diets. However, I also make clear that merely following my dietary recommendations is not enough. We must all try to understand why and how what we eat and where we purchase food are factors that have profound impact upon our personal and collective health freedoms. Therefore, I urge everyone to read at least one or two books on nutrition by a scientifically credible, 21st Century author. In the reception room of our clinic, a variety of contemporary nutritional works are available for patients to read as they wait for an appointment. We even loan those books to people who begin reading in the office and want to finish reading at home. Sometimes I buy multiple copies of important new books and give them to inquisitive patients and trainees.

Many women and men who read even one of those books finally begin to see the light. They change their diets because they begin to understand for themselves the types of foods that cause us to store fat year after year. A high percentage of them succeed in reducing excess body fat and achieving better health. Unfortunately, many other patients do not quite connect all the dots. They may find 21st Century nutritional texts to be a little too complicated or a little too detailed. Others just do not find sufficient motivation to change their old 20th Century beliefs or alter their ingrained eating habits and addictions.

Recognizing the enormous disconnect between what up-to-date, honest, 21st Century nutritional research tells us we <u>should</u> eat and what most of us actually <u>do</u> eat, I feel compelled to help bridge this gap. Having read and reread so many contemporary nutritional research works, I understand how many readers become overwhelmed by technical terminology, complex details, and foods that require hours of preparation. This book, therefore, is my attempt to summarize *essential* dietary information from several of the most prominent nutritional writers of the 21st Century. Of course, they do not all agree on every specific dietary recommendation. However, there is a strong consensus among most of these writers about the essential aspects of dietary habits and the prevention of obesity and other diet-related diseases. After summarizing the principles of excellent nutrition as presented in their works, I reduce the information further into an understandable dietary plan of action featuring simple menus and easy recipes. The culmination of this process is "**The Two-Page, Pro-Active, Strength for Life®, Every-Single-Day, Eating-For-Well-Being Guide**", a very focused, no-nonsense, two-page distillation of specific: (1) foods we should eat nearly every day; (2) foods we may eat occasionally and/or in limited quantities; and (3) foodstuffs we should eliminate completely from our diets.

In addition to summarizing the history of nutritional and dietary advice in the US starting in the last half of the 20th Century, I offer this work to accelerate the *American Diet Revolution!* I hope reading the summary makes you angry and motivates you to take personal action every day. This revolution, however important, is a quiet revolution, one we carry out by reading, by reflection, by discussion, by questioning "authorities," and by thoughtful dietary actions in our kitchens, at our local farmers' markets, in our food co-ops, and throughout our local communities. These actions are not as difficult nor as dangerous as the actions taken by the original American Revolutionaries, the colonists who risked everything to create a free country over two centuries ago. Today, we are revolting against a different type of colonization, one created by deliberate misinformation and sustained by those entities whose profits are directly proportional to the percentages of us weakened by obesity and constrained by other diet-mediated diseases. These economic forces want the majority of us to remain as we are—overly fat, drug-dependent, helpless, diabetic colonists. However, by rejecting scientifically unsupported dietary propaganda, and by refusing to purchase and eat foods we now know bloat and inflame our bodies, we can begin to rebel against these exploitive forces. In so rebelling, we choose to deploy peaceful, spiritual, and intellectual weapons of self-defense bequeathed to us by the authors of the Declaration of Independence, the US Constitution, and the Bill of Rights. Without realizing it, by purchasing and eating foods that enhance human well-being, each of us is enlisting as a soldier in the fight for health freedom—the *American Diet Revolution!*

Author's Note

Throughout this book, I capitalize "C" in the word "Century" when it is preceded by an ordinal number designating a specific 100-year span, such as "21st Century." I do this because it is appropriate in printed English to capitalize specific historical periods, such as "Renaissance" or "Stone Age." It is my contention that the 20th Century and the 21st Century are highly distinctive historical periods in this dietary context. Each of these centuries harbors specific historical events, social movements, economic shifts, environmental trends, and other unique characteristics that distinguish it from the other—and from all previous centuries as well.

The distinctiveness of the historical periods we call centuries was crystalized for me in the early 2000s. In a phone consultation with my daughter Caitlin, about a problem I was having with my computer, she asked, "What web browser are you using?" When I answered that I was using Internet Explorer, she exclaimed, "Dad, that's so 20th Century!"

By capitalizing "20th Century" and "21st Century," I am emphasizing the profound differences in how dietary advice was offered and received during these two periods. During the 20th Century, we accepted most nutritional information from "official" sources without questioning the origins, truthfulness, or methods used in gathering that information. It was an era of passive acceptance. Although the 21st Century has barely begun, it has distinguished itself already by our constant search for and review of the truthfulness of the information we encounter. We no longer accept "official" dietary information without questioning the integrity of its sources. Because of staggering advances in access to information during the current century, we are now capable of freeing ourselves from groups and organizations that previously controlled our access to foods by controlling our access to information about those foods.

Disclaimer

An essential principle set forth in this book is that prior to making any changes in his or her dietary or nutritional habits, each reader should communicate personally with at least one healthcare professional knowledgeable in the field of human nutrition. The present work advances general guidelines for healthful eating. It does not represent a dietary prescription for any one specific individual. The author assumes no liability for such personal use. All persons who read and plan to use information and dietary advice presented in this book should also discuss their diets and health with their personal physician(s).

Chapter One

Fighting for the Freedom to be Lean and Healthy

I t is no secret. We Americans have been losing a crucial war for the last 60 years—our fight to be lean and healthy. No matter what our financial standing, no matter what our country's military might, we are not a strong nation of free and independent people, if:

- more than two-thirds of us are obese or pathologically overweight, as we are today;
- the rate at which we use prescription drugs doubles in the next 20 years—as it has during the past two decades; and
- we continue to be increasingly dependent upon pain-killers and other drugs to slog through our days.

Ironically, for several decades most of us have realized that eating better foods and exercising are two critical elements in the fight to overcome obesity and related diseases and regain our health. We've responded by exercising more regularly and vigorously, as evidenced in recent years by geometric increases in the numbers of health clubs, bike trails, yoga classes, and women's and girls' sports opportunities. We've also tried valiantly to follow what we believed to be expert dietary advice. And yet, despite our growing exercise commitments, more and more of us are becoming obese and drug-dependent every year.

So, why are we failing?

If it is not due to a lack of exercise, could it be dietary mistakes are causing us to become obese and more vulnerable to obesity-related chronic diseases?

What can we do to reverse our negative trends towards obesity and increasing dependence upon drugs?

What can we do to win this war, to restore our personal and national health independence?

The first two major purposes of this book are (1) to examine those questions thoroughly and (2) to propose specific, practical actions each of us can take to reclaim our personal and collective health freedoms. This is not a war that can be won with mild protests. To recapture control of our well-being, we must engage ourselves actively and forcefully in the fight against large, entrenched economic groups that, to this very day, continue to profit from our passive acceptance of misleading nutritional advice and dietary propaganda.

The quality of the foods we eat and how successfully our bodies break down and assimilate the nutrients of those foods are two of the most important factors in our quest to achieve whole-body leanness, excellent health, and vibrant energy. Researchers have shown that the greatest exercise program in the universe cannot even begin to compensate for a diet dominated by foods:

- that disrupt and inflame the human gastrointestinal system;
- that upset the intricate balances of hormones and microbes in our bodies; and
- that—by raising our blood sugar levels rapidly and repeatedly— cause us to store excessive amounts of fat in our cells.

We must teach ourselves which foods we can eat to become leaner and healthier and which foods we must eliminate because they cause obesity, inflammation, and chronic disease. We cannot continue to blindly rely upon misinformation spewed out by those who profit most when we are disabled by obesity.

The third major purpose of this book is to summarize the most credible, scientifically based, up-to-date, and responsibly reported dietary and weight-loss information available today. This is not a simple task. For several decades, the field of nutrition has been—and continues to be—a minefield of conflicting dietary advice. Foods or nutritional products announced as beneficial for human health one year are denounced as toxic the next. If I had to describe with one word the state of clarity in the areas of nutrition and weight-loss advice, it would be "confusion."

Since the 1950s, nutrition and dietary advice have been dominated in the public domain by individuals and groups who have exploited and continue to exploit our confusion. Some of these people and groups of people merely have taken advantage of golden economic opportunities without considering consciously the origins or consequences of those opportunities. Many others, however, have purposely manipulated statistical data to achieve academic acclaim, realize enormous profits, or acquire immense influence and power. In doing so, they have deliberately subverted the scientific method—the organized process by which our civilization endeavors to advance knowledge. As long as intellectual confusion and deliberate deception continue to dominate the fields of agriculture, nutrition, diet, and health care, these sinister forces—

referred to collectively hereafter as **the Exploiters**—will retain an astounding degree of influence on and control of our health, our well-being, and, therefore, our personal freedom.

Why We Are Failing

To comprehend how we arrived at our present state of dietary health and dependence, we must briefly review the history of nutritional research and advice in the US from the 1950s through the first two decades of the 21st Century. Only by studying the origins of current mainstream dietary recommendations can we begin to understand the staggering extent of the misleading nutritional information we were subjected to in the last half of the 20th Century. By reeducating ourselves, we realize that the diverse array of severe chronic diseases we suffer from with great frequency—such as, Alzheimer's, diabetes, gastrointestinal disorders, autism, and ADHD—are direct consequences of following that deceptive dietary advice. When we learn that, by following scientifically unsupportable dietary recommendations, we were hoodwinked into making life-health-and-death nutritional wrong turns in the 1950s, '60s, and '70s, we cannot help but be disgusted. When we discover it was well-known amongst honest researchers by the 1970s that these recommendations were harmful to human health—and that the same dietary and medical advice continues to this day—it is infuriating!

Without follow-up action, intellectual fury can be self-consuming. To end the power and control of the Exploiters, to overcome their continuing thirst for profits at any cost, we must channel our anger into a peaceful form of guerilla warfare. That is, we must focus our energies by revolting in a civilized but forceful manner against the status quo. By educating ourselves, and by making personal dietary changes, we begin a strategic fight to regain not just our good health, but our individual and collective liberties as well.

What Can We Do?

Fortunately, since the year 2000, two seemingly unrelated revolutions of information have gained momentum. First, many highly capable and brave researchers and writers in the fields of nutrition and health have published honest studies and thoroughly-documented books exposing the deceptive methods used by the Exploiters in the last half of the 20th Century to gain control over what we eat and what we think about what we eat. These contemporary authors question why the scientific method was not utilized consistently by so many of their predecessors in nutritional research during those five critical decades. Backed by real clinical studies, they document extensively the direct physiological connections between many of our rising health epidemics and the prevailing dietary advice offered during this period and, sadly, still being offered today. From their careful reviews of the actual raw data—not merely whitewashed summaries—from research, we learn precisely how the results of many supposedly scientific studies were distorted deliberately rather than interpreted honestly. By reading the works of these contemporary authors, we begin to see how the dietary needs of human beings were not and are not congruent with most of the economic interests of the Exploiters. That education inspires us to then establish new personal eating habits that promote our health and well-being rather than the wealth, prestige, and power of those who would exploit us. It is only by doing this that clarity can triumph over confusion and each of us can achieve greater understanding of diet and nutrition in America.

In the second revolution of the 21st Century, the star of contemporary information dissemination—the Internet—has gone supernova. The tactics used by the Exploiters to suppress public disclosure of the falsehoods they spread in the last half of the 20th Century no longer work. The uncensored reach of the Internet exposes readily and thoroughly those dyspatriots who have cheated, lied to, stolen from, and otherwise violated the rights and well-being of Americans whom they should consider to be not their indentured servants or their colonists, but rather, their fellow human beings.

For most of us, the information summarized in the following chapters of this book is unsettling. We learn how we have been betrayed by persons, organizations, government agencies, and other entities which, up until now, we thought could be trusted. We see clearly why regaining control over our food supply requires not just protest, but a concerted revolution. To this day, the Exploiters, their obedient accomplices, and their organizations still dominate governmental committees, the media, medical advice, and nutritional academia. However, when our muskets are fully loaded with more truthful nutritional knowledge than we ever had in the past, we can reclaim much of the freedom, power, and control we trustingly, involuntarily, and, yes, ignorantly surrendered to the Exploiters during the last half of the 20th Century. Once we commit ourselves, enlist in the fight for honest dietary information, a third revolution, the *American Diet Revolution* will have begun.

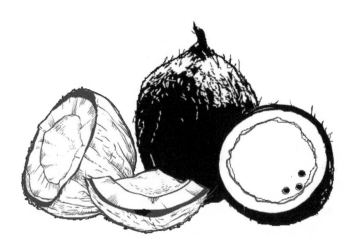

Chapter Two

A Brief History of Nutritional Advice Since the 1950s: Dietary Colonization

To study this period of nutritional advice in greater depth, I urge you to read ***Good Calories, Bad Calories*** (2007), ***Why We Are Fat*** (2010), and ***The Case Against Sugar*** (2016) by Gary Taubes and ***The Big Fat Surprise*** (2014) by Nina Teicholz. These works provide unbiased and uncensored historical reviews of how and why we Americans surrendered unwittingly our freedom to eat foods which help us to be lean and healthy. Being so misled, we became nutritional colonists, our diets dominated by industrial foodstuffs that make us sick, but enrich, empower, and embolden the Exploiters even to this day. Now, however, we finally have the knowledge and power to restore our health freedom.

In the 1950s, health care professionals in the US were concerned that the rates of heart disease and death by heart attack—which were thought to be relatively low in 1900—appeared to have increased dramatically during the first half of the 20th Century. In retrospect, as demonstrated by Taubes in ***Good Calories, Bad Calories***, much of what appeared to be an increasing rate of heart disease was due to faulty interpretations of incomplete data collected during the early 1900s.

From 1900 to 1950, the average life span of an American increased from 48 to 67 years, due primarily to improved public health measures (such as cleaner drinking water) and the discovery of antibiotics, resulting in fewer premature deaths due to infections. Furthermore, the invention of the electrocardiogram in 1912, the emergence of cardiology as a medical specialty in the 1920s, and the introduction of arteriosclerotic heart disease as a diagnosis in the International Classifications of Disease in 1949 were all major factors in creating the perception that the incidence of heart disease in Americans was rapidly rising.

During the 1950s, many health "experts" were not aware of those factors. They knew heart disease was the leading cause of death. They were determined to discover its causes and to propose solutions. Searching among several possible causes, some of those experts hypothesized that changes in the typical American diet from roughly 1900 to 1950 were the primary cause for the increasing prevalence of heart attacks and cardiovascular pathology. Relying again on misinterpretations of sketchy data, they were misled into believing that typical Americans at the end of the 19th Century were eating a lot less meat and animal fats and considerably more fruits and grains than average Americans in 1950. As Gary Taubes demonstrates, systemic misinterpretation of misinformation gave rise to false conclusions. Nevertheless, in the race to be first in curing heart disease, several "researchers"—whose work, by sheer coincidence, had been underwritten by such disinterested parties as Big Sugar—were inspired to reach the uninfluenced conclusion that the increasing consumption of dietary fats was the major cause for what they thought was an increasing prevalence of cardiovascular disease.

From this Petri dish of misinformation in the 1950s, one leading researcher emerged. Ancel Keys' research at the University of Minnesota had been supported since the 1940s by generous philanthropic donations from the sugar industry. He became the undisputed heavyweight champion of the hypothesis that saturated fats were the primary dietary cause for the increasing incidence of cardiovascular deaths and disease. His hypothesis seemed plausible to others because autopsies of many people who had died of coronary disease revealed fatty streaks in their blood vessels and heart tissues. Keys' unbiased opinion was that these fatty streaks were proof that dietary fat was a direct cause of atherosclerotic plaque, high cholesterol levels, and heart attacks. His opinion became known as the **Diet-Heart Hypothesis (DHH)** but was, in reality, the **Diet-Cholesterol-Heart Hypothesis (DCHH)**.

Within the upper ranks of the sugar industry, this hypothesis could have been dubbed "Fat Chance." Attracting attention to the idea that fat was the culprit diverted public attention from considering more likely suspects, such as sugar and grain-based foodstuffs that behave like sugar. Roman writer and patriarch Cicero had referred to this tactic 2,000 years earlier as "throwing dust in the eyes of the jury."

We were dusted.

Due to the continuing prevalence of heart attacks—most notably of President Eisenhower—the media and the public embraced Keys' proposal quickly and without demanding substantiation. Anxious to capitalize on his momentum, Keys set about to confirm his hypothesis with research studies, most of which were epidemiological in nature, that is, based upon his statistical analyses of written surveys of large groups of people. Very few actual, controlled, physical clinical trials were undertaken. Real research was expensive, time-consuming, and difficult to control. Time was a-wasting. People had to be saved from heart disease now. Therefore, based almost exclusively upon "selected" epidemiological studies, and without any real clinical evidence, Keys wrote and spoke extensively about how his research supported his hypothesis. He became the darling of an anti-saturated-fat and anti-cholesterol campaign, even to the point of being pictured on the front cover of a noted national magazine.

So great was Keys' popularity and influence that for decades most American researchers, academics, dieticians, physicians, politicians, and ordinary citizens continued to accept his Diet-Cholesterol-Heart Hypothesis fully, without bothering to question the lack of corroborating clinical evidence to substantiate it. Any honest dietary researcher who dared point out discrepancies in Keys' work or who proposed a different hypothesis was silenced quickly by Keys and his ardent supporters.

Today, in the world of real scientific research, there has been intense scrutiny of Keys' work, resulting in serious criticism of the decidedly unscientific methods and faulty conclusions he reached from his "research." Taubes' and Teicholz's reviews of Keys' works reveal clearly that the raw data in many of his studies does not support—and in some cases directly contradicts—the conclusions he reached and publicized.

In his "studies," the scientific method of evaluating research data was subverted. Much of the information from Keys' "research" was deliberately or inadvertently misinterpreted to support his Diet-Cholesterol-Heart Hypothesis. Nevertheless, in 1961, based on the supposed validity of Keys' hypothesis, the American Heart Association (AHA) published dietary recommendations to Americans that told them to significantly reduce their consumption of fats and, instead, eat higher quantities of carbohydrates—especially grains, but also fruits and vegetables. Keys himself was the guiding member of the AHA committee who wrote those guidelines. Even today, although we know those misleading guidelines were based upon falsified research, most Americans continue to follow them.

In the 1950s and '60s, no other researcher was able to receive sufficient attention in either academia or the media to question publicly Keys' analytical methods. Keys and his army knew in their hearts that he was right and were certain that their advice was what the American people needed.

To support their view that everyone should believe in the Diet-Cholesterol-Heart Hypothesis, Keys and his apostles continued to interpret research data in their own special way. For example, in one epidemiological study of 22 European countries, Keys reported and interpreted only the data from the six countries that supported his view. He omitted the data from the other 16 countries that did not support the Diet-Cholesterol-Heart Hypothesis. A few brave researchers at the time pointed out the fallacies in Keys' selective approach to the data; however, they were ignored. Once again, Taubes' and Teicholz's reviews of raw data from this entire study reveal how the scientific method was deliberately subverted to promote a hypothesis that could not be honestly substantiated.

To further establish the "truth" of the Diet-Cholesterol-Heart Hypothesis, those in the Keys camp used their falsely acquired prestige and power to crush support for any alternate or opposing hypotheses. Researchers with differing views—such as those who suggested that sugars rather than fats were the primary dietary cause of heart disease—were shouted down and even spat upon at what were supposed to be scientific conferences. These non-Keysians often discovered that their applications for grants to continue their research work were turned down or they were no longer being appointed or reappointed to positions in government agencies or to prestigious professional boards and committees.

For example, in 1957, the American Heart Association issued a report criticizing the Diet-Heart Hypothesis. Not to be refuted, Keys and one of his devoted supporters managed to get themselves appointed to a subsequent AHA committee which, in 1961, issued a new AHA report recommending to Americans that they could reduce their risk for heart disease by lowering the total amount of fat in their diets and eating polyunsaturated vegetable oils instead of saturated fats.

In researching her book, Teicholz interviewed some of Keys' contemporary researchers—most of them now elderly and retired—who dared to speak out against the Diet-Cholesterol-Heart Hypothesis during the last half of the 20th Century and suffered career setbacks as a result. Their personal stories are chilling to anyone who believes in the scientific method, freedom of speech, and academic integrity in the United States. In short, these independent thinkers were bullied into silence and academic oblivion. Adherence to the scientific method was replaced by the dogma preached by Keysians who knew they were right and knew they could use their nutritional righteousness to save the American people—not only from the epidemic of heart disease, but from the rising tide of obesity as well.

The Coronation of the High-Carbohydrate, Whole-Grain Diet

Over the next few decades, and in the disguise of nutritional certainty, Diet-Cholesterol-Heart Crusaders fanned out across the country to spread their good word. From positions of influence in governmental agencies and on academic committees, buoyed by "research" awards from Big Sugar, and with the unquestioning accompaniment of the media in the 1960s, '70s, and '80s, these apostles rose to prominence within organizations such as the American Heart Association and the National Heart Institute. Once established in positions of influence, these infiltrators issued dietary recommendations that Americans cut down on their consumption of fats, especially saturated animal fats, and instead eat more grains, vegetables, and fruits. Not to be outdone, the United States Department of Agriculture surged to the forefront of this holy army. With the 1992 publication of their crowning achievement, the Food Pyramid, the USDA was anointed Pharaoh of the Heart-Healthy, Whole-Grain, High-Carbohydrate Diet. At that time, very few people asked—and even today very few people ask—obvious questions.

Why should an agency created to oversee the production of agricultural crops have the unbridled power, unbiased expertise, and ultimate authority to advise citizens of the nation about what they should eat?

Does it follow that what is good for profits and production in the agricultural industry is necessarily healthful for humans to eat?

What are the backgrounds and credentials of the individuals who sit on the committees of the USDA and make these recommendations? Are these individuals serving truly in the health interests of citizens, or do they have stronger relationships with well-funded special interest groups?

In 1992, with little to no resistance, the USDA Food Pyramid became the golden model which all Americans—especially schoolchildren and their parents—were advised to follow when choosing foods to eat. It was reassuring to know that we were doing the right thing for our health, exactly what Keys and his entourage wanted. In reality, by following an unsubstantiated diet-health hypothesis, we were shackling ourselves with ignorance, obesity, and illness. Even today, many of us remain in the handcuffs and ankle irons of disease as a consequence of following the commandments engraved on tablets in the tomb of the USDA Food Pyramid.

What Happened When Americans Followed Recommended Low-Fat Diets?

At the time in which the official-sounding, low-fat, dietary recommendations were first issued in the 1960s and '70s, we Americans were not aware that those recommendations were based upon an unsubstantiated hypothesis. We believed we were being told the truth, that we could reduce our risk for heart disease if we ate less foods high in fats (such as eggs, butter, cheese, and meats) and more foods that were predominantly carbohydrates (especially breads, cereals, and pasta, but also fruits and vegetables). During the four decades after those guidelines became widely known, we: reduced our consumption of dietary fat by approximately 25 percent; substituted vegetable oils and synthetic fats for animal fats like lard and butter; drank skim and low-fat milk instead of whole milk; increased our intake of fruits and vegetables by more than 15 percent; and increased our intake of grains, cereals, and breads by almost 30 percent. We complied obediently with what the AHA, NHI, USDA, our doctors, and most dieticians recommended. We transitioned ourselves from a diet in which fats were the greatest source of calories to one in which carbohydrates reigned.

On the surface, these "official" recommendations made sense. We believed "experts" who told us that eating foods with fat and cholesterol would lead directly to clogged arteries and make us gain fat weight. And since one gram of a fat food has twice as many calories as one gram of a carbohydrate food, switching from fat foods to carbohydrate foods reduced the number of calories we were eating and, therefore, helped us lose weight, right?

Let's talk about that a little bit. There are only three primary sources of calories in foods: proteins, fats, and carbohydrates. When a dietary recommendation is made to significantly reduce our consumption of one of those three macronutrients, we must either reduce the total number of calories we eat each day or add calories from one or both of the other two sources. In the case of the holy Food Pyramid, the recommendation was that fat consumption be reduced drastically and carbohydrate consumption, especially grains, be increased significantly.

At the base of the Food Pyramid, the foundation of the USDA diet, was the recommendation that every American eat 7-11 servings of grains each day. According to the USDA Pharaoh, grains were the Elite Forces in the dietary war against heart disease, cholesterol, and obesity. On the second level of the Pyramid was the next most important branch of the army—fruits and vegetables. Meat and dairy foods, primary sources of proteins and fats, were relegated to the third level, symbolizing the Truth Squad's opinion that these were the main dietary causes of heart disease and obesity and reinforcing the idea that we should eat much less from these groups than we had in the past.

In the sandstorm that swirled around the Great Pyramid of 1992, very few of us were aware that it had been constructed of materials derived almost entirely from highly questionable interpretations of epidemiological studies rather than from honest evaluations of actual, physical clinical trials. Stated bluntly, there was almost no empirical evidence to support the recommendations that we should eat from each of these three food groups in the ratios depicted in the Pyramid. During those years, relatively few, truly scientific researchers asked questions such as:

What, if any, are the physiological effects when human beings consume 60-70 percent of their calories from carbohydrate foods—especially grains—each day?

How do different types of foods affect human blood sugar levels? For instance, do vegetable carbohydrates affect blood sugar levels in the same way as grain-based carbohydrates? Table Sugar? How do proteins and fats affect blood sugar levels?

Are there any negative health consequences if an individual's blood sugar rises precipitously or remains elevated several times each day?

Do any of the recommended foods have a direct negative effect on human tissue? For instance, do such foods cause indigestion or inflammation of the human gastrointestinal system?

How do fats affect our hormone levels? Carbohydrates? Proteins?

These are a few examples of the types of qualitative questions that could have and *should have* been asked and researched thoroughly before the Low-Fat, High-Carbohydrate diet was advanced as a cure for heart disease, diabetes, and obesity. However, Exploiters such as Big Sugar used their financial clout to guarantee that those questions did not receive much public attention in the last half of the 20th Century. Those in a position of influence already knew what was right. They did not need to ask scientific questions or follow scientific methods. They knew the truth. All we—their docile and obedient colonists—had to do was follow their advice. They were leading us out of the hell of heart disease and obesity and into nutritional health paradise.

Today, questions such as those offered earlier are just a few among hundreds that should be considered by any one of us who gives or accepts dietary advice. Epidemiological statistics, even when interpreted honestly, are useful primarily for considering broad concepts in nutrition and health. They are not by themselves sufficient to formulate specific dietary recommendations. We are not test tubes. Substances we ingest not only interact with each other, but also cause complex physiological reactions within our organ systems. If we really want to understand how foods affect our health, we need to examine closely and test carefully the complex physiological responses in our bodies when we eat, digest, and assimilate different types of foods.

Maybe things weren't—and still aren't—as simple as the Keysians, the AHA, the NHI, the AMA, the USDA, and others preached. At that time, however, they did not ask questions; nor did most of us.

How Did the High-Carbohydrate, Low-Fat Diet Affect Our Health?

According to epidemiological statistics of the US Center for Disease Control and Prevention, during the first four decades following the proclamation of the low-fat high-carbohydrate diet by the AHA in

1961, we Americans complied with the recommendations for drastic changes in our diets. We lowered the amounts of fat we ate. Instead of eating primarily saturated animal fats, we switched to "vegetable" oils and trans fats. We kept our protein consumption about the same, but we substituted chicken for beef, egg fakers and egg whites for whole eggs, and non-fat or low-fat milk for whole milk or cream. As our calories from fat declined, the percentage of calories from carbohydrates in our foods increased dramatically, especially from grains, of which we consumed about 30 percent more than before.

In addition to reforming our diets, many of us followed two other "expert" recommendations to prevent heart disease. Many of us started to exercise regularly by walking, biking, canoeing, and dancing more than we had in the first two decades after World War II. Just as significantly, the percentage of us who were smokers declined by approximately 33 percent.

With such a strong degree of compliance to the dietary, exercise, and tobacco guidelines proclaimed by distinguished authorities, you would expect dramatic improvements in our health. We anticipated especially that the rates of heart disease, death by heart attack, and obesity would decline greatly.

At first glance, some statistics appeared to show marked improvement. Between 1961 and 2001, the percentage of Americans dying from heart attacks declined significantly. The average total cholesterol of Americans also declined by almost 40 percent. However, a closer and more complete examination of the statistics from this era yields a very different evaluation of our health.

When we look a little closer, the decreasing death rate by heart attack was attributable primarily to improvements in and increased use of blood pressure medications and to the development of advanced life-saving emergency procedures, such as balloon angioplasty and heart valve transplants. The incidence of heart disease (without fatality) actually increased, as evidenced by a 470 percent increase in heart-saving hospitalizations during this period. **Any** increase in heart disease was very disheartening. The reduction in the percentage of smokers alone, independent of dietary factors, should have caused a corresponding decline in the rate of heart disease.

The statistics on cholesterol appeared to be just as perplexing. Study after study during this period demonstrated that the drastic dietary changes proposed by the AHA in 1961, and endorsed later by the NHI, AMA, and USDA, had little or no effect on lowering total cholesterol levels. It was only cholesterol-lowering drugs, introduced in the 1980s, that were causing decreases in total cholesterol levels. However, this was also a deceptive statistic because no independent, honestly performed, clinical studies from this era could demonstrate that lowering total cholesterol levels decreased one's risk of developing heart disease. Yet, still today, based primarily on arbitrarily determined high total cholesterol levels, many doctors—and ubiquitous television ads—continue to recommend cholesterol-lowering drugs to prevent or reduce the risk of heart disease. This is an excellent example of how misinformation in the last half of the 20th Century continues to compromise our health today. Without clinical proof that it is beneficial, Exploiters still acclaim the cholesterol-lowering effects of breakfast cereals and statin drugs to reduce one's total cholesterol. As Dr. David Perlmutter reveals in *Grain Brain*, real research today shows that low levels of total blood cholesterol may actually indicate an increased risk for developing dementia.

Two particularly troubling uses of a patient's total cholesterol level on a routine blood lipid test are to (1) declare his or her increased risk of heart disease and (2) to justify the prescription of an anti-cholesterol drug. Ironically, there is information on a standard blood lipid test that does correlate with the risk of heart disease. If a patient's triglyceride level is elevated, and/or HDL (high-density lipoprotein) level is low, his or her risk for heart disease *is* actually increased. Conversely, if that patient's triglycerides are low and/or HDLs are high, he or she has a decreased risk for heart disease. So why are these levels not the ones that doctors discuss with their patients routinely? Could it have anything to do with the fact that no drug has yet been developed to raise HDL levels? Here are some points we must consider:

- Total cholesterol levels can be lowered with drugs.
- Total cholesterol levels have been shown to have little or nothing to do with the incidence of heart disease.
- Total cholesterol levels are the most commonly cited statistic used by doctors for the prescription of drugs to lower serum cholesterol.
- Income to pharmaceutical companies from the sales of cholesterol drugs approaches one trillion dollars per year.
- The side effects from the use of cholesterol-lowering drugs are significant, often leading to the prescription of additional medications to counteract these side effects.

Does anyone else think there might be connections here? Is it subversive to question if such ongoing practices benefit the Exploiters greatly and affect the rest of us adversely?

Another measurement of the standard blood lipid test often used to justify the prescription of cholesterol-lowering drugs is the level of LDLs (low density lipoproteins), sometimes referred to as the "bad cholesterol." However, as Dr. David Perlmutter details in **Grain Brain** and in **Brain Maker**, numerous clinical studies over the past several years have shown clearly that one type of LDL carrier molecule, the so-called large, light, and fluffy LDL, is actually needed for normal function of the human brain. Deficiencies of this type of LDL molecule are associated with serious brain disorders, most critically with Alzheimer's Disease and other forms of dementia. Therefore, it would not be to a patient's benefit to use a drug to lower his or her total LDL level if the reason LDLs were elevated was because he or she had high amounts of the beneficial, large, light, fluffy type. And yet, routinely today, high total LDL levels, like total cholesterol levels, are used to justify prescriptions for cholesterol-lowering drugs with many known, negative side effects. This tragedy is compounded by the fact that, since the early 1990s, there has been a laboratory test which can be used to differentiate between beneficial, large, light (pattern A) LDL molecules and detrimental, small, hard, dense, oxidized (pattern B) LDL molecules. Unfortunately, only highly progressive physicians order and utilize this differential test. If this test were utilized more often, there would be far fewer prescriptions written for cholesterol-lowering drugs. To make the situation even worse, the foods that contribute the most to the formation of detrimental, small, hard, pattern B, oxidized LDL molecules are those which cause frequent, rapid increases in our blood sugar levels. Foods that raise our blood sugar levels are the foundation of the high-carbohydrate, whole-grain diet endorsed first by the AHA in 1961, beatified by the USDA, and recommended routinely still today by most physicians, dieticians, governmental agencies, etc.

In the last few paragraphs, my primary reasons for reviewing the effects of the low-fat, high-carbohydrate diet upon heart disease and cholesterol levels were to demonstrate: (1) that this diet failed to reduce heart disease; (2) that this diet has never been shown to reduce the levels of the harmful type of cholesterol carrier molecules (LDL pattern B); and (3) that, although drugs subsequently did reduce total cholesterol levels, this specific reduction alone did not reduce the incidence of heart disease.

And yet, in spite of a mountain of clinical evidence demonstrating that these methods were and are totally ineffective, this diet and these drugs remain the most commonly recommended treatments to prevent heart disease. Clearly, factors other than science *must* be responsible for the continuing use of these failed methods.

Rumblings of Revolution

By the early 1990s, it was clear to many honest researchers and health care clinicians that the Diet-Cholesterol-Heart Hypothesis was false.

Some scientists, especially in Europe, were brave enough to start firing at it directly. One of the first volleys came from Dr. Uffe Ravnskov, a Scandinavian physician and researcher who published *The Cholesterol Myths* (title translated) in Swedish (1991). Of course, those who were in control of nutritional information in the US ignored him, as evidenced by the 1992 publication of our beloved Food Pyramid.

Because there had been no confirming study to support the low-fat, high-carbohydrate diet recommended in 1961 by the American Heart Association, in 1993 a new study was launched to "prove it." The National Heart, Blood, and Lung Institute (formerly NHI, the National Heart Institute) allocated $725 million for the Women's Health Initiative, a study which would last 10 years. A group of 49,000 women, many of them overweight or obese, participated. In the experimental group, 20,000 women were instructed to reduce the amounts of eggs, butter, meats, and other fats in their diets. The remaining 29,000 women, the control group, were instructed to continue eating as they had before. The women in the experimental group complied with the instructions and cut their total fats by 22 percent and their saturated fats by 25 percent.

In 2006 and 2007, the 10-year results of the Women's Health Initiative were published in the *Journal of the American Medical Association*. The reports of this study revealed that the participants in the low-fat group were no less likely than the control group to have: breast, colon, ovarian, or endometrial cancer; strokes; or heart disease. Regarding obesity, in 10 years on a low-fat diet, in which they had also cut their daily caloric intake by nearly 500 calories, those in the low-fat group did not lose a statistically significant amount of total body weight. In addition, because their average waist circumference did increase significantly, the women in the low-fat group experienced a substantial increase in body fat. In sum, contrary to what the sponsors of the study expected, a large clinical trial confirmed what several smaller studies and many honest researchers had been saying for more than 30 years: the Diet-Cholesterol-Heart Hypothesis was false. A low-fat, high-grain diet did **not** reduce the rates of either heart disease or obesity.

During the 10 years of the Women's Health Initiative, critics of the Diet- Cholesterol-Heart Hypothesis did not wait idly for the results. By the year 2000, reports from many different dietary research projects throughout the world were causing objective researchers to question why and how the DCHH myth continued to dominate dietary advice and health care in the United States. At the same time, here in the US, epidemiological data from the Center for Disease Control and Prevention demonstrated that in the 40 years immediately after the AHA's recommendation of the low-fat diet in 1961: (1) the rate of diabetes in the US had risen from less than 1 percent to more than 11 percent and (2) the rate of obesity had increased from approximately 14 percent to 33 percent.

What was wrong?

Does this data prove that not only was the Diet-Cholesterol-Heart Hypothesis a failure in regard to heart disease but, even worse, that it was and is a cause of obesity and other serious diseases? After all, a fundamental maxim of health care is Hippocrates' warning: "First do no harm."

It would be easy to leap upon the old Keysian bandwagon trick of employing epidemiological statistics to claim absolute truth. To do so, however, would be to act as greedily, cowardly, irresponsibly, and dishonestly as those who advanced the Diet-Cholesterol-Heart Hypothesis in the second half of the 20th Century. Epidemiological data can only establish associations; it cannot demonstrate causality. In the next paragraph, we consider an example.

In the 1960s, the organic food movement began to emerge from relative obscurity. Its rise to prominence roughly aligns with the rise in obesity and diabetes rates in the US during the same period. If we were to use logic equivalent to what the Keysians used to advance the Diet-Cholesterol-Heart Hypothesis, we could claim that eating foods raised without artificial chemical fertilizers, herbicides, and other industrial enhancers causes obesity and diabetes. What such an epidemiological hypothesis would be lacking, of course, is a clinical trial comparing two randomly selected groups of people, one group eating organic foods and the other eating non-organic foods. In such a study, we could take physical measurements to determine if any specific, measurable health differences resulted over a period of time. For instance, if we measured the percentage of body fat of all participants in both groups before and after the clinical trial period, and we kept all other possible variables equal for each group, we might be able to substantiate the hypothesis that one diet produced a healthier body fat percentage or that there was no difference.

A clinical trial as described above is precisely what was never performed successfully with the Diet-Cholesterol-Heart Hypothesis prior to its coronation. It was advanced from a level of association to the altar of absolute truth without facing the scrutiny of the scientific method. It went virtually unchallenged for decades and unfortunately continues to dominate nutritional and medical advice in this country today. However, dominance gained under false pretenses is usually exposed eventually. In the first two decades of the 21st Century, that exposure occurred at a gradually accelerating speed, primarily due to the work of several new revolutionary authors who demand that the scientific method be restored as the way we determine the relative truthfulness of nutritional, dietary, and health care advice.

In the last half of the 20th Century, we allowed ourselves to be led blindly down a trail more lethal than a dead end; it was and remains a path to illness and to the unconscious surrender of our personal and collective freedoms. We should have demanded a much higher level of confirmation before we allowed ourselves to be led away. Our journalists, our politicians, our medical providers, and we ourselves lacked the fortitude to defend some of our most precious liberties—the freedoms to ask questions, to be healthy, and to be non-addicted. The 21st Century, however, is a new historical period, an age in which we have the information and the opportunity to revolt against those profiteers who have colonized us by obesity and other chronic diseases since the 1950s.

Most revolutions begin with a few leaders who see and speak out against deceitful practices and outright injustices in human societies and who inspire those around them to take action to make life better. In the fields of nutrition, dietary advice, weight loss, and health care since the year 2000, many new leaders have emerged—authors, doctors, and researchers—who have exposed the untruths of the 20th Century and provided us with accurate information and compelling incentives to reclaim our health and independence.

Dietary and Nutritional Information 2000-2017

In 2000, with the help of a publisher in Great Britain, *The Cholesterol Myths* by Uffe Ravnskov, M.D. was published in English and began to receive the wide readership it deserved. The first shot in the *American Diet Revolution* had been fired from abroad. Systematically, Ravnskov exposes the deliberate deceptions behind the unsubstantiated claims used by the Keysians to sanctify the Diet-Cholesterol-Heart Hypothesis and justify their cruel dietary and pharmaceutical experiments upon the American people. We in the United States were the unwitting guinea pigs in that experiment then; now we are the unhealthy victims of its disastrous results. The Exploiters gained wealth, power, and prestige. We gained fat weight, developed diabetes, increased our rates of heart disease, gastric reflux, and dementia, and lost many of the liberties enjoyed by those with good health. The Exploiters became our emperors, controlling us with addictive, destructive foods and drugs. We became their subjects—colonists dependent upon their highly industrialized food and drug commodities.

In this country, the first bugle call of the *American Diet Revolution* was sounded in 2001. In an article in **Science** magazine, entitled **"The Soft Science of Dietary Fat,"** Gary Taubes details the deceptive tactics employed for decades by those who wanted the Diet-Cholesterol-Heart Hypothesis to reign supreme regardless that facts were to the contrary. Not merely a critic, Taubes reintroduces us to an alternative hypothesis, researched extensively in Germany and Austria in the 1920s and '30s, that hormonal imbalances, especially of insulin, were the primary drivers of obesity and possibly heart disease as well. In 2002, Taubes followed up with an article entitled **"What If It's All Been a Big Fat Lie?"**, published in *The New York Times Magazine*. Taubes had issued the dietary equivalent of the Declaration of Independence.

From the work of Ravnskov and Taubes, a picture began to emerge as to why the Diet-Cholesterol-Heart Hypothesis did not (and still does not) stand up to scientific scrutiny. Its ardent supporters had failed to consider the physiology of human digestion. The Keysians had assumed, without clinical evidence, that fat and cholesterol in foods simply made their merry way directly into our arteries and hearts, around our organs, and onto our hips and waists. They did not consider (or perhaps were influenced by their Sugar Daddies not to consider) that when human beings consume foods, complex physiological reactions are triggered in all organ systems. Instead of real clinical research, they relied almost exclusively upon statistical data which, when it did not meet their needs, they could manipulate to agree with their preconceived opinions and the desires of the Exploiters who supported them. At last, early in the 21ˢᵗ Century, the weaknesses and deceits of their arguments were being exposed.

In 2004, the next direct strike against the Diet-Cholesterol-Heart Hypothesis was launched from England. Dr. Natasha Campbell-McBride, a British physician and nutritionist, published *Gut and*

Psychology Syndrome, a detailed clinical work demonstrating the complex interrelationships between our diet, our digestive system, our nervous system, and our health. From her descriptions at the cellular level, we begin to understand how certain foods—especially grain-based foodstuffs—cause direct damage to the mucosal lining of the gastrointestinal (GI) tract. Such extensive tissue injury to the GI tract not only causes extreme digestive disorders such as gastric reflux and Crohn's Disease, but also leads to neurological diseases as diverse as autism, ADHD, schizophrenia, and depression.

Dr. Campbell-McBride describes in great detail the natural dietary methods used in her clinic for many years to help patients heal from damage to their GI tract and, thus, recover from the diseases such gut disorders cause. She provides extensive menus she uses to help individuals regain GI health, as well as precise information regarding foods that must be avoided. In addition, she offers many recipes for health-fostering foods that can be prepared economically at home.

Campbell-McBride's work is a sterling example of a new breed of physician, well-versed in the scientific method, knowledgeable of current research, and dedicated to helping her patients heal without unnecessary medications. She is also one of the first authors to introduce us to the microbiome, the vast herd of microorganisms lining the GI tract in each one of us, the health and proper function of which relates directly to our overall health and function. Although most of her clinical research is original, she also pays tribute to some of the earlier researchers whose work was overlooked or lost in the Diet-Cholesterol-Heart stampede during the last half of the 20th Century.

In 2007, Gary Taubes published *Good Calories, Bad Calories*, a meticulously documented and remarkably comprehensive work in which he details nutritional theories and practices dating back to the 19th Century. Thanks to Taubes, we are able to place the era of the Diet-Cholesterol-Heart Hypothesis into the context of nutritional research and dietary advice over the past 150 years. From this perspective, we clearly see how false assumptions and unscientific reasoning by biased individuals and groups led directly to the dietary disasters in the last half of the 20th Century. We also learn about the leading scientific researchers of the 1920s and '30s in Germany and Austria. Those researchers were in the midst of demonstrating the differing hormonal effects of specific types of foods, particularly that diets high in certain concentrated carbohydrates cause an excessive release of insulin, which, in turn, causes the body to store and hoard fat. Unfortunately for us, in the social upheaval before and during World War II, those researchers were dispersed or killed, and their pioneering work was lost.

After World War II, the fields of nutrition and diet were dominated by a new group of individuals who were much more interested in statistical epidemiology, promoting their own pet ideas, and the financial causes of their supporters, than in performing and studying actual clinical research. Taubes thoroughly documents how pride, prejudice, and money, rather than the scientific method, prevailed in those fields for over six decades. Perhaps the greatest contribution of his work is that Taubes demands we consider the most crucial dietary factor in obesity, diabetes, and heart disease: eating foods that cause our blood sugar levels to rise rapidly and repeatedly, causing the secretion and release of the hormone insulin, which, in turn, initiates a cascade of unfavorable pathological events in our bodies.

In 2008, Dr. Campbell-McBride fired another rocket in the battle for nutritional honesty and better cardiovascular health by publishing ***Put Your Heart in Your Mouth***, a powerfully succinct frontal attack on the Diet-Cholesterol-Heart Hypothesis. She repeats Ravnskov's demand that the scientific method be restored as the process by which we judge the truth or falseness of any hypothesis. In the first chapter, she lists and summarizes dozens of studies which demonstrate conclusively that the Diet-Cholesterol-Heart Hypothesis could not be and is not true. Then, as in *Gut and Psychology Syndrome*, she takes us down to the cellular level to understand the pathological processes of atherosclerosis and heart disease.

Campbell-McBride's detailed discussion and descriptions of heart disease and its causes stand in stark contrast to the shallow, epidemiological arguments presented by the supporters of the Diet-Cholesterol-Heart Hypothesis, such as the authors of *The China Study*, which was published in the same year (See Denise Minger, *The China Study*: **Fact or Fallacy**). Campbell-McBride proposes rational and affordable dietary changes we can all make to liberate ourselves from the colonies of disease created by following the misguiding advice of the Keysians. To truly understand scientific studies, she urges fellow physicians to read clinical research reports in their entirety rather than rely only upon one-paragraph summaries that are often misleading. Finally, she leads us back to the microbiome, the vast colonies of bacteria that inhabit our GI tract and that we depend on for good health. She provides us with a mouth-watering array of natural foods, such as sauerkraut, that are rich in beneficial bacteria and we can prepare economically at home. In addition, she cites the physiological reasons why our diets should include ample amounts of unpolluted saturated fats. For decades and without any evidence, the Keysians and Exploiters told us to avoid saturated fats. Today, growing numbers of well-executed clinical studies tell us that some saturated fats from "clean" sources are, in fact, essential for good health.

In 2010, Taubes scored another direct hit on the Titanic-like Diet-Cholesterol-Heart Hypothesis with the publication of *Why We Get Fat*. Whereas *Good Calories, Bad Calories* is a heavily referenced work which is sufficiently detailed for health care and science professionals, *Why We Get Fat* is pragmatic and accessible to the general reader. In a straightforward manner, he addresses and exposes many of the myths and misconceptions in nutrition and dietary advice which fueled the astronomical increases in the rates of obesity and diabetes during the last half of the 20th Century and which continue to fatten, sicken, and confound us in the 21st Century. Perhaps most importantly, he helps us understand: why calorie-restriction diets and exercise-only programs are not effective methods to prevent or reverse obesity; why saturated dietary fats do not necessarily make us fat; and why foods that raise our blood sugar levels—especially concentrated carbohydrate foods—do cause us to store excessive levels of body fat.

During the last four decades of the 20th Century, in response to the American Heart Association's recommendation that we reduce the amount of fat and increase the amount of carbohydrates in our diets, we Americans complied by raising our daily consumption of grains and cereals by 30 percent. In 2011, cardiologist William Davis launched a new missile at those recommendations with the publication of *Wheat Belly*. In this myth-shattering book, Davis provides direct insight into a major cause of the GI injuries Dr. Campbell-McBride described years earlier in *Gut and Psychology Syndrome*. His breakdown of the components in modern wheat helps us understand why wheat raises our blood sugar levels faster than table sugar and, therefore, causes the frequent and intense insulin responses which Taubes describes in *Good Calories, Bad Calories* and *Why We Get Fat*.

Central to the main hypothesis of *Wheat Belly* is Davis's description of the extreme methods used by technicians of the grain industry in the 20th Century to alter the traditional wheat plant and thereby increase per-acre yield. Their goal was to increase the volume of seeds—the only part of the plant humans can eat—and decrease the susceptibility of a plant to damage by insects and mold. In the 1940s, they achieved this primarily through cross-breeding plants with the characteristics they were seeking. When those methods were not sufficient, grain researchers resorted to more "advanced" methods in the 1950s and '60s to alter the genetic makeup of wheat, such as exposing experimental plants to x-rays or strong chemicals. The results of those efforts were new hybrids of the original wheat plant, hybrids that had much greater seed volume and were resistant to mold and insects. Unfortunately, the effects upon the GI tracts of the human beings destined to eat those altered wheat seeds were not considered. One such alteration, an increased concentration of a super carbohydrate called Amylopectin A, causes a human's blood sugar level to rise much faster and higher than when she or he eats unaltered wheat. As Taubes and others had already documented, foods that cause our blood sugar levels to sharply increase trigger the release of insulin, the hormone expediting the storage of body fat and initiating several other negative health processes.

Davis describes a second major change in the genetic makeup of modern wheat that is just as dangerous to human health as Amylopectin A. The drive for increased productivity resulted in alterations of the proteins in wheat, especially of gluten and one of its protein components, gliadin. Many of these altered proteins are partially or totally indigestible by humans and, thus, putrefy in the small intestine where they cause direct damage to the cell wall and the junctions between these cells. In **Wheat Belly**, Davis identifies several of the precise substances in grain-based foodstuffs that cause the bowel diseases which Dr. Campbell-McBride had described in detail several years before.

In the works of Ravnskov, Campbell-McBride, Taubes, Davis, and many other writers seeking dietary honesty during the first decades of the 21st Century, a common theme emerges. The experimental alterations of grains beginning in the 1940s, the Diet-Cholesterol-Heart Hypothesis of the 1950s, and the unquestioning support from influential health organizations throughout the remainder of the 20th Century, created tremendous economic opportunities for well-positioned groups and individuals. The economic interests of those groups and individuals were mutually beneficial. As Americans ate more grain, the grain industry—Big Farma—became more profitable. As we ate more and more grain, more of us became obese, diabetic, and prone to a multitude of chronic diseases. This guaranteed greater demand for more goods and services in the health care industry, the Medical Industrial Complex (MIC), and in the pharmaceutical industry (Big Pharma). Collectively, these three groups are the leading Exploiters. As 21st Century nutritional writers for freedom all proclaim, the Diet-Cholesterol-Heart Hypothesis and the "Eat Healthy Whole Grains" myths flourished then—and continue to flourish today—primarily because they present easy opportunities for immense profits. The Exploiters will do all they can to preserve their current economic advantages by extending those myths as far into the future as possible.

In *Wheat Belly,* Davis provides detailed documentation of the severely negative consequences to human beings who eat modern, wheat-based foodstuffs. Obesity, diabetes, GI diseases, and heart disease are only a few of those consequences. Davis reminds us that the glycemic index of wheat is higher than that of table sugar. Eating two slices of organic whole wheat bread raises one's blood sugar level as much as eight teaspoons of table sugar, triggering a sustained insulin reaction. From the thorough work of Taubes, we understand that the repeated release of insulin to lower our blood sugar levels accelerates pathological processes that result in obesity, diabetes, and heart disease.

In 2013, with the release of *Grain Brain*, neurologist David Perlmutter deepened our understanding of the detrimental consequences of eating a high-carbohydrate diet featuring an abundant amount of grains. Although wheat is the most toxic of the modern, genetically-altered grains, all grains cause extensive damage to the organ systems of the human body, most frighteningly, perhaps, to the nervous system. Perlmutter details many of the systemic pathways to neurological diseases, from headaches to Alzheimer's, that are caused by eating foods that raise our blood sugar levels. Frequent spikes in blood sugar levels, such as those which occur after eating grain-based or high-sugar foods, accelerate the pathological process of glycation in which sugar molecules bond with and alter the structure of proteins. These abnormal proteins—called glycoproteins—can no longer fulfill their normal and important physiological functions. For example, these abnormal proteins can cause shrinkage in the size of functional tissue in the human brain by accumulating as non-functional, space-taking, cellular debris known as Advanced Glycation Endproducts (AGEs).

Perlmutter reminds us that in 1994, both the American Diabetes Association (ADA) and the American Heart Association (AHA) recommended that 60-70 percent of our diet should come from carbohydrate foodstuffs. Not coincidentally, from 1997 to 2007, the rate of diabetes doubled in the US. He also informs us that being a diabetic doubles a person's risk of developing Alzheimer's Disease. Those statistics are good news to the ADA and the AHA because they ensure that the services of their organizations and its members are going to be in greater demand in the future as more Americans become colonized by heart disease, obesity, diabetes, and dementia. As Perlmutter explains, the cost to all of us for providing advanced health care to so many totally disabled patients will bankrupt our already depleted system of health insurance. If, in 2013, we were not yet certain of the serious health problems caused by kneeling at the altar of the false Diet-Cholesterol-Heart Hypothesis, *Grain Brain* convinced us that we must rise up and revolt against this thoroughly discredited hypothesis.

In 2014, our understanding of modern nutritional science, politics, and dietary advice took a major step forward with the publication of *The Big Fat Surprise* by journalist Nina Teicholz. Based upon a nine-year detailed study of the actual raw data and complete reports of nutritional research from the 1940s to the present, as well as personal interviews with surviving researchers, she reconstructs the history of nutritional science, governmental and institutional involvement, and public acceptance of dietary advice during that period. Through her faithful and objective recounting, we see precisely how Keys and his followers manipulated epidemiological data to advance their cherished Diet-Cholesterol-Heart Hypothesis, despite the fact that they had no direct clinical evidence to support it. In reading her personal interviews with nutritional scientists from both sides of the issues, we learn how Keys, by force of his personality alone, was able to dominate their field of study for decades.

After summarizing virtually all of the important dietary research from 1950 to 2013, Teicholz presents some of the logical conclusions that can be developed from an honest review of that work: (1) the Diet-Cholesterol-Heart Hypothesis has never been substantiated; (2) the high-carbohydrate diet, which its followers managed to force upon the American people, has resulted in unprecedented increases in serious chronic diseases; (3) the continuing prevalence of this diet has no basis in science but, instead, is due primarily to the immense profits being realized by certain vested groups; and (4), contrary to the propaganda tunes being played still today, real research demonstrates that human beings need to be eating some of the types of fats, even some saturated fats, that the American Heart Association, the American Diabetes Association, the American Medical Association, Big Sugar, and other financially motivated entities have led us to believe—and continue to try to convince us—are unhealthy.

As stunning as the revelations of dietary research deception during the last half of the 20th Century are, from Teicholz we learn something even more astounding. Even in 2014, the committee in charge of writing the updated guidelines for official dietary advice of the US government remained dominated by persons who supported the discredited Diet-Cholesterol-Heart Hypothesis. Therefore, we are forced to consider that the fraud of the 1950s and 1960s may still be continuing today. It will require a great deal of strength and perseverance—a revolution—to free ourselves from domination by the Exploiters (Big Farma, Big Pharma, and the Medical Industrial Complex) and their entrenched surrogates.

In late 2014, William Davis advanced our understanding of nutrition, health, and the physiology of human digestion with the publication of his second revolutionary book, **Wheat Belly Total Health**. A practicing cardiologist, Davis was very disappointed in his rate of success, not only in helping his obese cardiac patients, but also with his own health. Despite the fact that he had been running three to four miles per day, several days a week, for years, he was a significantly overweight diabetic. In his blood work report, his triglycerides were an extraordinarily high 350 mg/dl and his HDLs an abysmally low 27mg/dl. Through intensive study of nutritional and dietary research, he concluded that his high-carbohydrate, low-fat diet, replete with large amounts of grain-based foodstuffs, was the major cause of his obesity and diabetes, as well as that of many patients in his practice. By first eliminating wheat products and then all other grain-based foodstuffs from his personal diet and from his dietary recommendations to patients, both he and they began to decrease their body fat and recover their health. In his own case, not only did he shed many pounds of excess body fat, but his triglycerides fell from 350 to a healthy 42 mg/dl and his HDLs increased from 27 to a robust 97 mg/dl. He was no longer a diabetic colonist! Many of his patients achieved similar results. Based upon his direct personal and professional experience, and his ongoing study of nutritional and digestive physiology, Davis developed his grain-free, total-health program.

Among several outstanding achievements in **Wheat Belly Total Health**, two are particularly important to the *American Diet Revolution*. First, Davis contributes mightily to our understanding of why eating grains causes so many serious GI problems, from indigestion, bloating, and gas to irritable bowel syndrome, gastric reflux, "leaky gut," and celiac disease. He accomplishes this with a thorough explanation of digestive physiology, a topic never addressed by the Keysians or by the big grain-eating advocates of today.

Cows, ruminants that thrive on eating grasses in the classification Poeceae, have GI systems well-suited for eating and utilizing the nutrients from these plants. They have four-compartment stomachs; secrete 100 quarts of saliva per day; grow up to 100 sets of adult teeth in a lifetime; chew, swallow, regurgitate, chew their cud, then swallow again; and have short spiral intestines highly populated with the types of bacterial flora that allow them to digest and absorb nutrients from entire grain plants without developing bowel obstructions.

In contrast, humans have one-compartment stomachs, secrete only about one quart of saliva to aid digestion each day, have only one set of adult teeth that are ground down by the gritty abrasiveness of grains, do not chew a cud, and have long, loopy intestines in which incompletely-digested, grain-based foods can lodge and putrefy for days. In addition, we can only partially digest the seeds of grasses and, even then, only after those seeds have been highly processed—pulverized, cooked, or subjected to other powerful agents to break them down before we attempt to eat them. In short, our GI systems are not designed to chew, swallow, digest, and absorb the nutrients from grass seeds such as wheat, rice, corn, oats, barley, rye, etc.

For the first 190,000 years of human existence, our Homo Sapiens ancestors did not eat grass seeds. It was only about 10,000 years ago that we began to eat those seeds in significant amounts. Although we developed the skill to cultivate these grain plants, which made possible the permanent population centers we call cities, we still did not have the capability of digesting the seeds of Poeceae easily or well. As a consequence, eating those grains leads to an extensive number of GI diseases, a problem which has been compounded geometrically by the agricultural scientists of Big Farma, who have altered the genetic makeup of these plants frequently and extensively over the past 70 years. The grass-seed foods our great-grandparents ate 100 years ago are very different from those grown and marketed today. Even organically-raised grains are significantly altered, which is compounded by the nearly uncontrollable factor of cross-pollination in agriculture.

To our understanding of diet, digestion, health, and disease, a second major contribution made by Davis in ***Wheat Belly Total Health*** is the identification of specific components in grass seeds (wheat, barley, rice, corn, oats, rye, etc.) that cause specific problems for humans. In other words, Davis does not merely shoot from his hip and claim that eating grass seeds does this or that. Rather, he identifies known intrinsic elements of these seeds, describes many of their pathological effects when they are eaten by human beings, and cites specific clinical research studies in which laboratory measurements are used to affirm these effects. That is to say, he functions as a responsible clinical scientist and physician.

We must take a moment to contrast Davis's work with the biased and unscientific epidemiological methods applied by Keys and his followers in the 1950s and '60s and with the cowardliness of those researchers who have failed to stand up for honest research in the decades since. Davis explores how lectins, a type of protein abundant in grains, has detrimental effects upon the human digestive system. One type of lectin in wheat is known as Wheat Germ Agglutinin (WGA). In all grain plants, lectin proteins are highly resistant to mold, fungus, and insects in the field. Because of these attributes, agricultural scientists have manipulated modern grains to have much higher concentrations of lectins than they did 75 years ago. Greater resistance to molds, fungus, and pests means greater yield per acre and greater profits for the grain industry. Unfortunately, those scientists neglected to consider if the increased concentrations of lectin proteins in grains would have any adverse effects upon the human beings who eat them.

Clinical research demonstrates that WGA and many other lectins are almost completely indigestible for human beings. In addition, many of these proteins are so tough they cannot be altered by most external methods, such as cooking, baking, or fermentation. Therefore, when grain foods with lectins are eaten, these undigested proteins congregate and putrefy in the small intestine, where they cause damage to cell walls and the microvillae (the minute, hair-like structures through which many of the nutrients in foods are absorbed into the bloodstream). WGA increases the permeability of the small intestine, meaning many undigested or partially digested proteins, substances which should not enter our blood, gain entrance. Once those abnormal proteins gain access to the bloodstream, they trigger many serious inflammatory disease processes, including blood clots, autoimmune diseases, celiac disease, and dysfunction of the pancreas and gall bladder. Some abnormal proteins in the bloodstream migrate to the brain where they cause neurological disorders such as autism and Alzheimer's Disease.

A second specific protein in modern wheat which Davis identifies is gliadin, a major component of gluten. Tests of seeds more than 100 years old reveal that gliadin was present only in extremely minute amounts prior to the 20th Century. However, as grain company scientists have increased the protein content of wheat through selective breeding and other methods, gluten and gliadin concentrations have grown substantially since the 1950s. Too bad no one considered the effects of gluten and gliadin upon the human GI tract. The relationship between gluten and celiac disease is well-known now. But as Davis points out, celiac disease and gluten sensitivity are just a small part of the story. More pervasive are the additional and seriously damaging effects of the specific gliadin portion of gluten.

In the small intestine of human beings, gliadin is broken down into smaller protein elements called peptides. Aided by increased intestinal permeability, these peptides leak into the bloodstream where they navigate to the brain and bind with opiate receptors, the same receptors to which morphine, heroin, and the drug Naloxone attach. The migration of gliadin to opiate receptors in the brain is responsible for the addictive nature of grain-based foodstuffs. After eating a bagel, a slice of bread, a muffin, or some other wheat-based food, we want to eat another. Clinical measurements verify that eating foods containing morphine-acting compounds such as gliadin causes human beings to consume an average of 400 kilocalories more per day than do members of a control group who do not consume foods with such compounds. In addition, studies show that the administration of Naloxone, a drug to combat heroin addiction, can prevent such excess consumption. This begs the following question. Which is the better method to prevent obesity: abstaining from foods with gliadin or taking the drug Naloxone?

Addiction to opiates is one of the most serious of contemporary health epidemics. In light of the clinical evidence compiled by the revolutionary writers and researchers of the 21st Century, we must confront a question that Big Farma, Big Sugar, and their friends do not want us to even consider: Is there a relationship between addictive, high-carbohydrate, grain-based diets and addiction to opiates?

Alpha-Amylase Inhibitors, allergens not present in ancient grains, constitute a third component of wheat and other grains that Big Farma technicians have bred into modern hybrids to reduce plant susceptibility to pests in the field and thereby increase crop yields. Unfortunately, as Davis demonstrates, these inhibitors are not only toxic to insects, but also cause allergic reactions in human beings, reactions ranging from sneezing, hives, diarrhea, eczema, and cramps to Wheat-Derived, Exercise-Induced Anaphylaxis (WDEIA), a potentially fatal reaction in wheat-eating athletes during moments of moderate to extreme physical exertion.

Phytates are a fourth major element of modern grains with demonstrably negative effects upon our health. Phytates are the storage form of phosphorous and are present in abundance in the fiber of nearly all modern grains. Big Farma has bred modern plants to have a high fiber content, which makes them sturdier in the field as well as more resistant to pests. In the human GI system, however, phytates bind with iron and zinc, which makes these minerals very difficult for humans to absorb. Tests show that eating as little as one to two ounces of oats, wheat, or barley can reduce our absorption of these essential minerals by 90 percent.

In **Wheat Belly Total Health**, Davis identifies several other specific components of grains that disrupt the human GI system and cause or contribute to a diverse array of health disorders, such as tooth decay, nervousness, irritable bowel syndrome, gastric reflux, and dysbiosis, an unfavorable alteration in the bacterial flora in the gut. However, one disease-causing effect of consuming grain-based foodstuffs towers above all others: the ability of grains to raise our blood sugar to high levels rapidly, repeatedly, and for prolonged periods of time. This undeniable effect can be easily measured by testing an individual's blood glucose levels before eating a particular type of food, 30-60 minutes after eating it, and every 30-60 minutes thereafter for two or more hours. Davis performed similar tests on some of his patients. Comparing blood glucose levels at each time interval for each different type of food affords the opportunity to compare the propensity for each food to elevate blood sugar levels. One cup of cooked oatmeal raises blood sugar levels as much as 11 teaspoons of sugar. Thus, we know that eating oats causes our blood sugar levels to rise very rapidly. Organic whole wheat toast raises our blood sugar levels even higher and faster, not only faster and higher than oats, but higher and faster than table sugar. Despite these findings, thousands of times per minute, whole wheat and whole oat cereals and breads are touted as being "heart healthy" in TV commercials by dieticians and doctors.

Some of the many detrimental consequences of repeated and rapid increases in blood sugar levels, especially as a cause of Type II diabetes, have been known for a long time. However, we understand more fully the health dangers of such surges in blood sugar levels when we read works like **Good Calories, Bad Calories, Why We Get Fat**, and **The Case Against Sugar** by Gary Taubes. In **Wheat Belly Total Health**,

Davis identifies the specific component of grains most responsible for raising our blood sugar levels: Amylopectin A.

Amylopectin A is a highly-concentrated carbohydrate stored in the seeds of grass that provides the energy to initiate sprouting, a function it fulfills magnificently in grain fields. In the human GI tract, its effects are equally spectacular. Unlike indigestible proteins in grains, such as Wheat Germ Agglutinin, Amylopectin A is broken down and absorbed very rapidly into the blood stream, causing a flash flood in blood glucose levels. During such surges of blood sugar, glucose molecules can combine with and alter the structure of blood proteins. The resulting abnormal (glycated) protein can cause inflammation, autoimmune disease, or become a type of biological debris that can accumulate in virtually any organ system of the human body. Known as Advanced Glycation Endproducts (AGEs), this debris remains in the affected organs permanently, causing inflammatory disorders such as cataracts, plaques in blood vessels and the brain, and osteoarthritic joints. This non-functional tissue interferes with the normal functions of the organs in which it is lodged permanently.

To summarize, in **Wheat Belly Total Health**, Davis identifies many of the precise components of grains that cause measurable abnormal reactions in the human body, reactions which lead directly to multiple forms of serious acute and chronic diseases. But Davis is not a negative writer or physician. As Natasha Campbell-McBride did 10 years before in **Gut and Psychology Syndrome**, Davis ends his book with a comprehensive eating plan to eliminate the grains that fatten and inflame our bodies and replace them with nutritious foods that help us to recover our health.

In 2015, with the publication of **Brain Maker** by neurologist David Perlmutter, our understanding of digestive physiology and the detailed effects of specific foods on the human GI system took another giant step forward. His previous book on the subject, **Grain Brain**, had been released only a few years before. However, so much new research information had been published in the interim, it was essential that Perlmutter update his findings and recommendations significantly in this new book.

The biggest explosion of new information regarding digestion during this time came from research of the microbiome, the vast worlds of microscopic organisms that cover our bodies—skin, nose, eyes, and ears— and dwell most abundantly in the human GI tract. Researchers have studied how these microorganisms, predominantly bacteria, interact with the cells in our gut as well as with the foods and other substances we ingest. To a much greater extent than was ever understood before, these interactions have profound effects upon our health, our ability to digest and utilize the nutrients in foods, our ability to fight and prevent potential diseases, and even upon our thought processes. Being a neurologist, Perlmutter focuses primarily on the relationships between the physiology of our gastrointestinal and nervous systems. However, he emphasizes strongly that the health and functions of all bodily systems are highly dependent upon the health of our gut and that of our microscopic partners in the microbiome.

In essence, we are all farmers with vast herds of microorganisms we must maintain in favorable proportions. Therefore, we must eat ample amounts of foods that sustain large populations of the types of bacteria beneficial to our health and minimize the ingestion of foods and substances that promote proliferation of the types of microbes detrimental to our bodily functions. If we succeed in raising herds of beneficial bacteria, not only do they optimize the physiology of digestion in the gut, they also defend us against potentially lethal invading organisms, such as viruses and virulent bacteria. In addition, if we eat the right foods and avoid toxic ones, our beneficial microbes, which thrive especially by digesting vegetable fibers, will produce essential nutrients, such as Vitamin B-12, as byproducts.

In short, the health of each one of us is inextricably related to the health of the microorganisms that live in the gut.

In **Brain Maker**, Perlmutter describes in detail how substances in certain foodstuffs not only disrupt the balance of our microbiota, but also cause damage to the cells lining our gut and to the connections between these cells, called tight junctions. Among the most notorious of those food toxins are gluten and wheat germ agglutinin, intrinsic components of modern wheat. Along with other substances in modern grains, these two toxins cause breaches in the gut wall, allow partially digested abnormal proteins and sugars to leak into the bloodstream, and, in turn, lead to autoimmune reactions, abnormal hormonal secretions, and neurological disorders ranging in severity from ADHD to autism to multiple sclerosis to Alzheimer's Disease and other forms of dementia.

One particularly outstanding feature of **Brain Maker** is the degree to which Perlmutter explains why and how the foods we eat affect the composition of our individual microbiomes. By microscopic analysis of fecal material, researchers can measure with accuracy the proportions of the bacterial species inhabiting each person's GI tract. By comparing the microbial populations in groups of individuals with certain disorders, distinctive patterns of the bacterial populations emerge among members of these groups when compared to individuals in control groups without such disorders. When we compare the degree of precise laboratory methodology utilized by contemporary researchers of the microbiome with the slipshod statistical methods employed deceptively by the Keysians, the USDA, and other disciples of the Diet-Cholesterol-Heart Hypothesis, we see clearly why the dietary and health advice of the 20th Century was so easily manipulated and became so detrimental to our well-being.

As two other physician/researcher/writers before him (Natasha Campbell-McBride and William Davis), Perlmutter does more than merely summarize research and demonstrate that eating certain types of modern foodstuffs is a primary cause of many devastating chronic diseases. Like Campbell-McBride and Davis, he emphasizes that not eating formerly traditional foods essential to human health, such as saturated fats, also increases our risk for developing such diseases. Therefore, in the last half of *Brain Maker*, he provides detailed menus and recipes by which we can begin to heal from the diseases caused by the dietary misinformation we have been bombarded with since the 1950s. Following his recommendations, we are guided away from highly-processed, grain-based foodstuffs and back to simpler traditional foods—such as raw greens, fermented vegetables, and healthy sources of fat—that enable each of us to nourish the microorganisms in our GI tract upon which our health depends.

In 2015, another major advance in our understanding of the role of the microbiome in human digestion came with the release of *Gut Balance Revolution* by endocrinologist Gerard Mullin. Mullin continues the now-established 21st Century tradition of writer/researcher/practicing physician turned revolutionary, as the title of his book proclaims. He, Perlmutter, Davis, Campbell-McBride, and Ravnskov stand in stark contrast to the obedient academic "researchers" and uninquisitive physicians who dared not question the Diet-Cholesterol-Heart Hypothesis during the last five decades of the 20th Century and who, in far too many cases, continue to follow and preach that falsehood today.

Mullin illustrates in detail the complex functions of the billions of competing microbes populating our GI tracts and elucidates how differing types of foods, drugs, and other substances affect the important balance between these competitors. He emphasizes how important diversity in our internal microbial environment is to our overall health, just as variety in the organisms of our external environment is to the health of our planet. For example, he explains that vegetables grown in composted organic soil are measurably richer in nutrients primarily because the medium in which they are grown—the microbiome of these plants—

has a more diverse population of beneficial microorganisms than the microbe-deficient soil of plants treated with insecticides, herbicides, and chemical fertilizers.

Based on his research and clinical experience with patients in his practice, Mullin presents a three-stage dietary program to restore balance to one's microbiome. He contributes especially to our understanding of obesity and successful weight loss. He proposes recovering our health, not just by changing our diets, but also by restoring balance to other aspects of our lives, such as sleep, exercise, and mental relaxation. In short, he presents a comprehensive approach to enjoying the daily activities of our lives and to liberating ourselves from colonization by obesity and related chronic inflammatory diseases.

Early in 2016, two books were published that proposed we Americans should increase dramatically the amounts of healthful fats in our diets to reverse colonization by obesity and disease and reclaim our health freedom. These works are *Eat Fat, Get Thin* by Mark Hyman, M.D. and *Smart Fats* by Stephen Masley, M.D. and Jonny Bowden, PhD. Then, in January of 2017, nutritionist and anthropologist Nora Gedgaudas released *Primal Fat Burner*, the most eloquent argument to date for the Paleo Diet. Gedgaudus reminds us that we human beings are who we are today because our ancestors—for more than 200,000 years—ate animals. During the past 10,000 years, as grains have replaced fats as our primary source of dietary calories, our muscles and brains have shrunk, our stores of body fat have increased dramatically, and we have become hapless, dependent victims of chronic, preventable, disabling diseases.

In the spring of 2017, heart surgeon Steven Gundry, M.D. released *The Plant Paradox*, a giant step forward in our understanding of how the foods we humans eat have profound physiological and pathological effects upon our bodies. Based on decades of experimental research, he focuses especially upon the pathological reactions caused by lectin proteins. Lectins are abundant not only in grain-based food products, but also in many other foods we have been told in the past are beneficial to our health. For instance, the lectin proteins in the seeds and skins of tomatoes, cucumbers, eggplant, peppers, and other vegetable-like fruits trigger major inflammatory diseases in many humans who eat and attempt to digest them. In addition, lectins are abundant in chia seeds, pumpkin seeds, and sunflower seeds. Rather than being "health foods," these seeds can cause damage to the GI tract and contribute to many serious disease processes.

In addition to challenging us to understand lectins, Gundry demands we consider carefully the quantities of fats and proteins in our diets. In regard to the Paleo and high-fat dietary movements, his message might be paraphrased as, "Hold on there! Let's not overdo it. Eating too much protein and too much fat—especially animal protein and saturated animal fats—also can be catastrophic for our health."

As do the other distinguished physician/researcher/writers of the 21st Century, Gundry offers highly detailed dietary plans and recipes to guide his readers through the new health science of eating for well-being. He demonstrates very clearly how we can replace some saturated animal fats with plant fats (such as from avocadoes, macadamias, and walnuts) and replace some animal proteins with plant proteins (such as from hemp seeds). *The Plant Paradox* is a major contribution to the study of human nutrition and health. In addition to providing a wealth of new scientific information, Gundry's work reminds us that, if we wish to enjoy the freedom of good health, we must study and question nutritional advice on an ongoing basis.

* * *

Since the 1950s, elite economic groups have dominated dietary advice in the US. By following their recommended low-fat, high-grain diet, we Americans have been colonized by increasing rates of: obesity; diabetes; neurological, gastrointestinal, auto-immune, and cardiovascular diseases; drug addiction; and several types of cancer. Continuing economic domination by the Exploiters is contingent upon perpetuation of their recommended diet.

Our health care "system" offers almost no financial incentives for an all-out effort to prevent obesity and other diet-related diseases. Instead, the greatest profits in health care are directed to industries devoted to the ongoing management of such diseases. A vast population of helpless victims receiving a constantly growing supply of drugs and in need of extensive and expensive medical services is where the dough is.

Let's face it. We are not a nation of healthy people.

More than two-thirds of us are obese or pathologically overweight. At these rates of colonization, even as the wealthiest nation in the history of the planet, we cannot afford health care for all citizens. The Exploiters are engrained deeply in the power structures of commerce, health care, government, and the media. No groups or entities of comparable size and influence are capable of fighting successfully on behalf of individual citizens.

So, let's do something about it ourselves!

Absent George Washington and the other founding patriots, our only viable means of breaking the bonds of colonization is guerilla warfare. By revolting individually and in small groups against dietary oppression, we can liberate ourselves from obesity, from preventable diseases, and from becoming overly dependent on drugs. The following chapters detail why and how there must be an *American Diet Revolution!*

Chapter Three

The Case for an American Diet Revolution

eginning in the 1950s, Ancel Keys and his followers advanced the hypothesis that the high frequency of heart disease and related deaths in the United States and other highly developed countries was due primarily to high-fat diets, which caused the buildup of cholesterol in the bloodstream, blood vessel walls, and the heart. Without clinical verification of this hypothesis, but with substantial support from the sugar, grain, and other industries, they recommended drastic changes to the American diet. Those recommendations were adopted by major medical institutions such as: the American Heart Association, the National Heart Institute, and the American Medical Association, and later by the US Department of Agriculture. Throughout the last half of the 20th Century, this hypothesis was advertised, supported, and promoted by virtually every major medical organization, pharmaceutical company, governmental health agency, and vested interest group. During the same period, this misinformation was reported dutifully and uncritically by all branches of the media. Those few honest journalists and researchers who did object to the unscientific methodology used to prop up this hypothesis were squashed into silence by Keysians who believed we should not question divine truths such as the Diet-Cholesterol-Heart Hypothesis. In the belief system of the Keys' tribe, the scientific method should be used only to evaluate hypotheses that had not been pre-ordained.

During the last half of the 20th Century, we Americans followed the dietary changes recommended by Keys' disciples. We ate much less fat, especially saturated fat, and substituted new types of commercially created fats, such as trans-fats, for old standbys like butter and lard. As we decreased our intake of traditional dietary fats, we increased our consumption of carbohydrates, especially from grains and other sugars, but also from fruits and vegetables. In addition, we followed the recommendations to stop smoking and exercise more. We were led to believe that making those lifestyle changes would improve our health and especially lower our risk for developing heart disease.

But how beneficial did the changes actually prove to be?

Subsequent clinical and epidemiological studies have affirmed that exercising more and smoking less have indeed helped us achieve very significant health benefits. However, the same claim cannot be made for the high-carbohydrate, high-grain, low-fat Keysian diet. When analyzed without bias, no long-term research study supports continued promotion of this diet or the Diet-Cholesterol-Heart Hypothesis.

A famous longitudinal study of lifestyle habits and health in the US is the Framingham Heart Study. On a regular basis for over 60 years, researchers have examined, questioned, and kept comprehensive physical statistics on a large group of citizens in a moderate-sized community in Massachusetts. Results from this comprehensive trial reveal no evidence that lowering total cholesterol levels in the blood lowers a person's risk of developing heart disease. Other results from the Framingham Study mirror the health statistics of the entire US population. Diabetes, which afflicted less than 1 percent of Americans in 1961, now cripples more than 11 percent of us. The prevalence of obesity, which was about 14 percent in 1960, is now more than 36 percent. Gastrointestinal diseases, cancers, and neurological diseases are also all substantially more frequent now than they were before the low-fat, high-carbohydrate diet was first recommended by "experts" (and then followed faithfully by those of us who failed to question it).

During the last half of the 20th Century, a few brave researchers, thinkers, physicians, and others did object to the continued reverence for a hypothesis that did not stand up to the scrutiny of the scientific method. Their voices were rarely acknowledged by those preaching, shouting, and riding on the Diet-Cholesterol-Heart bandwagon. Fortunately, in the first years of the 21st Century, a new wave of bold writers/researchers/physicians rose to challenge the perpetuation of the dietary dogma of the 20th Century. These writers demanded that the scientific method be applied fairly and openly to the Diet-Cholesterol-Heart Hypothesis. They have researched carefully how this hypothesis first arose, was advanced without real clinical trials, was propped up by the falsification of "confirming" data, and since then has been maintained as scripture only by the suppression of contradictory data. These writers have also proposed alternative hypotheses that are supported by actual clinical research and have put forth dietary recommendations based upon this supporting data. Furthermore, several of these writers are practicing physicians who have utilized their new dietary methods successfully with many patients in their practices for several years and documented their beneficial results.

So Why Does the Diet-Cholesterol-Heart Myth Continue to Reign Supreme?

If researchers in the 21st Century have demonstrated clearly that the Diet-Cholesterol-Heart Hypothesis is false and that the high-carbohydrate, high-grain, high-sugar, low-fat diet is causing increases in serious chronic diseases, a fair question is this: Why does this hypothesis still dominate medical practice and dietary advice in the United States?

Not surprisingly, the simple answer to this question is that the continuation of the Diet-Cholesterol-Heart Hypothesis myth is still extremely profitable for the Exploiters. The real answer, however, is power. The depths of deception and the extent of manipulation to which exploiting individuals and groups will go to maintain their prestige and power are as astonishing as they are infuriating. In reading Nina Teicholz's **The Big Fat Surprise,** we are stunned that, in the Age of Information, the Exploiters can still dominate our thoughts and actions so thoroughly by dietary misinformation and nutritional confusion. In each of our GI tracts, the foods and drugs the Exploiters manufacture, distribute, and recommend destroy the colonies of beneficial microorganisms upon which the health independence of every human being depends. In standing by idly, as passive Acceptors of their products and propaganda, we allow these Exploiters to take away our health freedom and perpetuate their domination. For as long as we continue to be fooled by their lies and to be weakened and sickened by their inflammatory foods and drugs, we are doomed to remain their loyal, dependent, colonial subjects.

The Diet-Cholesterol-Heart Hypothesis gave its creator an enormous boost in academic prestige and paved the way for lucrative careers for its supporters, especially its early supporters. Once this hypothesis began to receive notoriety, there was much to be gained for those who climbed on board Keys' train. Professorships, research grants, committee appointments, governmental agency positions, and other goodies were available to those who were the faithful passengers and became his ardent messengers. However, those were only the small players, merely convenient facilitators in this story.

The Profit/Health Dilemma

In the 1950s and '60s, soon after Diet-Cholesterol-Heart began to take hold, leaders of certain interrelated industries recognized and exploited the opportunity to expand their operations, profits, and influence. Of these opportunistic industries, the biggest, most profitable, and most powerful were and are: Big Farma, particularly the grain and sugar cartels; Big Pharma, the drug and petrochemical industries; and MIC, the Medical Industrial Complex. These three supremacist groups have gained immense power during the reign of the Diet-Cholesterol-Heart Hypothesis. Their insatiable appetites for more power and more money dictate their need to prolong this myth for as long as possible.

For Big Farma, the dictators of the world agricultural industry, grains and sugars are by far the most profitable commodity. More than 50 percent of calories consumed by humans throughout the world are from wheat, corn, and rice. It is staggering to think of the demand for products that, on average, every human being on the planet consumes in large quantities every day. Relative to most other types of food, grains are easy and cheap to produce, store, ship, process, and sell. Fruits and vegetables, by contrast, are more difficult to grow, highly perishable, and expensive to store and ship. Animal products are also expensive to raise, process, store, and transport. Therefore, Big Farma is all for perpetuating our current addiction to grain-based foodstuffs manufactured from seeds of grass.

In addition to being sold as raw commodities, seeds of grass are extremely valuable as the highly-transformed foods they can become. Humans cannot digest raw grass seeds. To become even partially digestible, the seeds must be processed extensively: pulverized, ground, and/or cooked in some fashion. Each layer of processing—milling, grinding, baking, packaging, transporting—presents yet another economic opportunity. For instance, the raw materials used for a loaf of bread may be 10 percent or less of the final $.4.00 cost at a store. All intervening steps of processing provide profits for middlemen, but little or no additional nutritional or economic value to colonists who pay for them. In short, highly-processed, grain-based foodstuffs—bread, muffins, bagels, chips, donuts, pizza, etc.—are a bonanza for Big Farma and its subsidiaries. For those of us who purchase them, however, these products are equivalent to buying our food at a coal company store. Not only are these overpriced products nutrient-poor and calorically rich, but they also contain inherent substances that cause serious health problems, as we learn from books such as **Wheat Belly Total Health**, **Grain Brain**, **Brain Maker**, **Gut and Psychology Syndrome**, **Gut Balance Revolution**, and **The Plant Paradox**.

The next great profiteer from the perpetuation of the Diet-Cholesterol-Heart Myth is Big Pharma. The USDA-endorsed, calorically-concentrated, nutrient-poor, highly-processed, grain-based, foodstuff diet—which most of us have been following for decades—has led to skyrocketing incidences of obesity, diabetes, cancers, neurological diseases, and other serious health disorders among those of us who are the current American colonists. This is great news for the pharmaceutical companies; they are well-prepared and very eager to fulfill prescriptions for those of us unfortunate enough to need the pills, potions, powders, and other elixirs they have designed to counter the effects of our unhealthy diets. They are just as excited to fulfill secondary prescriptions to counter the side effects of their primary potions, as well as tertiary medicines to counter the side effects and interactions of the first two; and it goes on and on.

The economic keys to Big Pharma's exponential profits have been the unparalleled increases in obesity and diabetes in the US over the last 60 years. Being obese doubles one's risk of developing diabetes. Once a person is colonized by diabetes, it is unusual for him or her to ever again be liberated from medication dependence. Not only are more of us becoming diabetics, but we are becoming diabetic at earlier and earlier ages. If a teenager becomes diabetic, it is likely that he or she will need diabetic medications for 50 or 60 years. Therefore, he or she is a much more lucrative profit center for Big Pharma than an adult who becomes diabetic at age 50 or 60. In addition, once an individual is colonized by diabetic medications, the probability increases that he or she will need additional types of drugs, which means additional profits and power for the pharmaceutical industry.

The drive for ever-greater profits and power are the primary reasons why the Diet-Cholesterol-Heart Hypothesis continues to dominate the American health care industries. This is the crux of the Profit/Health Dilemma. There is a negative financial incentive in our economy for citizens to be healthy. Treating diseases is extremely profitable. True health care—striving to prevent disease by nurturing well-being—is decidedly unprofitable, especially for the pharmaceutical industry.

The fewer people who are obese, the fewer people who are diabetic, the less profit and power for Big Pharma.

From the perspective of the pharmaceutical industry, each individual American is a potential profit center. The more medications each citizen needs, the more profit for Big Pharma. The longer that individual can be kept alive while using as many medications as possible, the greater the return on investment for Big Pharma. So why would they ever object to the dietary advice that grew out of the Diet-Cholesterol-Heart Hypothesis? From Big Pharma's point of view, the more people who are obese and diabetic, the better. Therefore, they love the status quo, the pro-inflammatory, high-grain, low-fat diet advocated by the USDA, AHA, AMA, et al.

> Just by coincidence, the profits from the sales of their statin drugs to lower cholesterol are especially fabulous. And be comforted, fellow colonists, they are working feverishly on more types of drugs to treat the symptoms of dementia and its related diseases, the next great frontier of pharmaceutical profiteering.

Without becoming cynical, we colonists must pursue another line of questions regarding the Profit/Health Dilemma. Several 21st Century writer/researchers—notably Perlmutter and Davis—have demonstrated why and how the high-carbohydrate, low-fat, high-grain diet is not only pro-inflammatory, but also addictive. If this is true, would it not be logical to ask if there is a possible relationship between this diet and another contemporary health crisis: the opioid epidemic? Let's consider three possible links.

First, as Davis, Gundry, and Perlmutter describe, certain grain proteins, such as Wheat Germ Agglutinin, cannot be broken down completely and digested in the human GI tract. Instead, these proteins putrefy and cause damage to the tight junctions between the enterocytes, the single layer of cells lining the small intestine. Rather than continue their normal digestive trip through the human gut, some partially digested proteins leak through the weakened junctions between the enterocytes and into the bloodstream, where they do not belong.

This is Leaky Gut Syndrome.

Once in the bloodstream, these rogue proteins migrate to various organ systems. Most notably, gliadin, one of the protein components of gluten in wheat, crosses the blood-brain barrier and binds to opiate receptors in the brain. The "high" human beings experience when these receptors are stimulated triggers our desire to seek similar stimulation from more food or other substances. This is just one example of how eating grains can create addictive behaviors.

A second link between high-grain diets and opioid addiction occurs when proteins other than gliadin leak through damaged tight junctions into the bloodstream and mate with excess glucose to form abnormal glycoproteins. These irregular sugar proteins do not break down in the human body but, instead, accumulate as cellular debris—Advanced Glycation Endproducts (AGEs)—in every organ system of the body, notably in the brain, muscles, and joints. The human immune system identifies AGEs as invaders and mounts an inflammatory response. In the brain, inflammation against accumulating debris interferes with the transmission of neural impulses. In our joints, AGEs cause and accelerate arthritis. In muscles, they cause myofascial pain. Chronic joint and muscle pain are the most common reasons opioids are prescribed. These habit-forming drugs are not curative and lose their pain-killing potency with repeated use for extended periods of time. An addicted colonist seeks increasing amounts of these drugs, placing a physician in the impossible position of trying to alleviate a patient's pain and, at the same time, trying to avoid addiction.

A third link between high-grain, fat-causing diets and opioids is the recent discovery that fat cells are not merely idle repositories of stored energy but are metabolically active, just like most cells in the human body. Fat cells secrete inflammatory chemicals that migrate to joints and muscles and cause or exacerbate pain syndromes. We seek whatever means of relief we can, which often leads to opioids. The greater our fat mass, the greater the amount of inflammatory substances we secrete. Because high-grain diets are a leading cause of obesity, they increase the risk of opioid abuse.

Therefore, it is reasonable to propose that the addictive and inflammatory high-grain, high-carbohydrate diet—promoted fervently by the Exploiters since the 1950s—has created not only the obesity and diabetes epidemics but, in addition, plays a major causative role in our current opioid crisis.

Let's talk about another diet-related arena of profit for Big Pharma, one that stems from the overuse of antibiotics in the US. It is well-known, of course, that such overuse has created many strains of pathological bacteria that have mutated to become resistant to nearly all antibiotics. Less known, however, are the cumulative negative effects of such overuse upon the beneficial microbes in the GI tracts of all of us who are helpless colonist-consumers. As Mullin, Perlmutter, Gundry, and Davis each describe, when an individual takes an antibiotic, sizable populations of "good" bacteria are wiped out just as surely as are the invading organisms for which the drug is targeted. As a result, the natural immune protection normally provided by our friendly microbial armies is diminished. As these authors also point out, approximately 80 percent of the antibiotics administered in the US are to livestock. So, those of us who consume foods derived from animals treated with antibiotics consume the residuals from these drugs. Such secondhand antibiotic consumption disrupts our microbiomes and increases our risk for obesity, diabetes, and other inflammatory diseases.

> Cha-Ching! Cha-Ching! Cha-Ching go the bank accounts of Big Farma and Big Pharma as we are colonized by their terrorists in our colons!

A very close relative of Big Pharma is the petrochemical industry. Increased grain consumption since the 1950s has meant vastly increased use of pesticides, herbicides, and chemical fertilizers. Significant residuals of these chemicals are then assimilated into the plants. When we humans eat these "conventionally grown" grain-based foodstuffs, we absorb some of these residual chemicals directly via our digestive systems. When poultry, livestock, and marine creatures are raised with chemically-treated grains, we absorb these chemicals secondhand by eating foods such as eggs, milk, meat, and fish from these contaminated animals. Whether we assimilate these chemicals directly or indirectly, they are detrimental to the beneficial types of bacteria in our microbiomes. As Gerard Mullin demonstrates in detail in ***Gut Balance Revolution***, whatever throws the herds of microbes in our gut out of balance has a decidedly negative impact upon our health. In this way, the petrochemical industry contributes mightily to our colonization by disease. Given the huge profits Big Petro reaps from our current grain-dominated diet, members of that cartel are also unlikely to work for anything other than preservation of the dietary status quo.

The third major Exploiter of economic opportunity created by the grain-based, high- carbohydrate diet is the Medical Industrial Complex (MIC). The explosion of the obesity-diabetes-addiction-dementia epidemic has made possible almost limitless expansion of medical services in the US. It has created opportunities for a host of providers and facilities: doctors, therapists, nurses, hospitals, clinics, emergency medical services, ambulances, medical equipment providers, nursing homes, rehabilitation centers, etc. Health care services and supplies now account for nearly 20 percent of the gross national product in the United States with all signs pointing to a continuing rapid increase in this percentage. Clearly, the severe health problems created by the prevailing American diet are accelerating a looming economic catastrophe. What happens when the cost of health care for us, the new American colonists, reaches 40 percent of the GDP in the United States?

More profits for the Exploiters? Or does the American colonial economy implode?

Most health care providers in the United States entered their respective fields out of a deep desire to help people be healthy. In making a career choice, many of us who are health care providers did not realize the extent to which the demand for our services would be dependent upon exponential increases in obesity, diabetes, and other diseases caused by the high-carbohydrate diet based on the false Diet-Cholesterol-Heart Hypothesis.

The reality is that obesity and related diet-caused diseases are the primary cause of the runaway expansion of health care needs and costs. The more of us who become obese, the faster and higher health care utilization will continue to rise. Conversely, if we Americans were to revolt against the status quo and begin eating in a manner that promotes health and leanness, there would be a decline in the demand for health care services. Many health care providers who were unwilling to change their approach would become unemployed. Hospitals and clinics that are now billing perhaps 50 percent of their services for obesity-related disease care would have to cut back on staffing and building plans. There would be a ripple effect, leading to contractions throughout the Medical Industrial Complex and its vast array of supportive industries. Clearly, from an economic point of view, it is far more lucrative for all members of MIC to go with the flow, to continue to support a diet and system that they can depend on for an unending supply of obese, diabetic, arthritic, addicted, and disabled patients who will need more and more services and more and more intensive care for as far into the future as one can possibly see.

The Profit/Health Dilemma is not a dilemma for MIC. There is far more money in cancer drug research and treating cancer patients after the fact than there will ever be in trying to reduce the dietary and environmental causes of cancer. Even more lucrative for MIC is the fast-expanding arena of care for the neurologically disabled. Continued dominance of the Diet-Cholesterol-Heart Hypothesis and the high-grain, high-sugar diet is paving the way for massive building and personnel expansions to care for the vast numbers of new patient-colonists with Alzheimer's disease and other forms of dementia.

The New American Revolutionaries

Despite the gargantuan power and influence of the Medical Industrial Complex, living within its borders is a subset of individuals who have the power to lead a revolt against its seemingly limitless exploitation of patients who have been and continue to be colonized by obesity and related diseases. These are the same individuals who entered their health care careers because they wanted to help people become healthy and enjoy remaining healthy. Many of these individuals now realize that much of their economic success is because so many patients are obese. Rather than continuing to profit primarily from the epidemics of obesity and disease, these health care professionals would prefer to see more people achieve better health, even if it means a slight decrease in their own personal incomes. These are orthopedic surgeons and physical therapists whose waiting rooms are dominated by patient-colonists who are 50, 75, or 100 pounds overweight and, as a consequence of their obesity, need a new knee, rehabilitation, then a new hip, rehabilitation, then another new knee, more rehabilitation, and so on. They are cardiologists, thoracic surgeons, nurses, and dieticians who have witnessed for years that patients do not succeed in losing weight on calorie-restricted, low-fat, high-carbohydrate diets and, as a consequence, continue to become diabetic and heart-diseased at increasing rates. They are chiropractors, like myself, who feel the accelerated deterioration in the spines of patients whose obesity-causing diets are overloading and inflaming their joints, muscles, and nervous systems. They are the dentists and hygienists who witness how phytates in grains erode the enamel of our teeth. They are pediatricians and therapists who note that nearly all autistic and hyperactive children have severe digestive disorders and who see firsthand the explosion of obesity in children.

These and so many other types of health care providers see their patients as they see themselves—not as perpetual dependents colonized by debilitating diseases, but instead, as unique persons who want to be as healthy and independent as possible. The vast majority of these health care providers are motivated by the gratification felt when a patient overcomes a disorder and takes all possible proactive steps to avoid being incarcerated by that disorder again in the future. The reality is that many of us providers have yet to identify the common denominator in nearly all contemporary diseases: the prevailing American diet. Therefore, I call upon all of us who are health care professionals to take the lead in the *American Diet Revolution!* We, as a group, enjoy the privilege of a thorough education in human physiology, allowing us to understand the nuances of contemporary research in digestive physiology. It is our responsibility as dedicated health professionals to help as many patients as possible to improve both their health and our own by: reading and learning the truth about nutritional research; applying newly acquired knowledge to what they and we choose to eat; and taking primary responsibility for maintaining their own and our own personal well-being. It is our duty to inspire our patients and ourselves to break the bonds of colonization by disease and reassert our rights to become as independently healthy as possible.

Certainly, I do not suggest all leaders of the American Diet Revolution must be health care providers. The impact of diet on our health is understandable to all people who are willing to read and think. At present, however, voluntarily or not, nearly all of us who are health care providers are members of the Medical Industrial Complex. We profit directly and personally from the obesity epidemic. We bear the primary responsibility to lead the revolt against the disease-creating Diet-Cholesterol-Heart Hypothesis.

Another challenge I issue specifically to every health care provider is to refuse to accept passively anything I have stated in this book. We do not need another legion of unquestioning followers, such as those researchers, physicians, dieticians, and others who surrendered their independence to the holy armies of Keys in the 1950s and beyond. Do not accept anything I say, any more than you should accept the prevailing dietary dogma that has been used to brainwash all Americans since the 1950s. Instead, I challenge you to read for yourself some of the books by the authors I have cited, to read a few of the original complete clinical reports they cite, to read works by other nutritional researchers, and to study complete clinical reports you discover along the way. Come to your own conclusions. Develop your own dietary advice, your own reading list, and your own way of applying your knowledge to the questions your patients ask and the concerns they raise. I am extremely confident that when intelligent people read a broad representation of the nutritional information available today, an overwhelming majority will see that the dogmatic dietary advice which has prevailed since the 1950s was—and continues to be—a cruel experiment on the citizens of our nation. This experiment has enabled several industries to realize enormous profits. During this period, the percentages of people in the US who are obese, diabetic, addicted, and suffering from dementia and other serious chronic diseases have risen nearly as fast as the profits in the industries that service those of us who have become diet-disabled. It is telling that heart disease, which should have decreased dramatically if the Diet-Cholesterol-Heart Hypothesis had been true, has not diminished during this time span, despite the fact that we are smoking less and exercising more. Furthermore, it is clear that the current opiate epidemic is an end result of the increased use of all types of painkillers to combat the pro-inflammatory, high-grain, high-sugar diet foisted upon an unsuspecting American citizenry.

Although it is essential for all health care providers to consider the causes of the increasing prevalence of disabling chronic diseases in the US, there are also much higher callings to all of us who are citizens of this country and inhabitants of this planet.

Our first calling, as Americans who enjoy the privileges of education in a free and democratic society, is to be vigilant about the threats to our freedom. It is our duty to question "authorities" and self-proclaimed "experts," especially when we suspect something they say or recommend may be wrong or unjust. In Germany in the 1920s, an insufficient number of citizens were willing to speak out as Hitler and the Nazis rose to power with dogma and then ruled the country through fear. Although fraudulent claims and practices in health care do not rise to the level of totalitarianism, the perpetuation of the Diet-Cholesterol-Heart Hypothesis has substantially weakened our nation and, therefore, our claim to liberty. A nation cannot be strong if two-thirds of its citizens are obese and/or pathologically overweight. A nation cannot be strong in the future if the rates of preventable mental health disorders, such as dementia and Alzheimer's Disease, continue to increase. When so many of us become disabled by preventable diseases, we become permanent colonists of the Exploiters and are no longer free citizens. Our nation was founded by colonists who risked everything to establish a free and independent republic and rid themselves of tyranny. It is the responsibility of each one of us now to free ourselves from the tyranny of those who have prospered economically while we the people are colonized by diseases caused by foods and other substances we should never ingest in the first place.

A second calling to each one of us is to protect Earth, an incredibly beautiful planet whose habitability for humans and other advanced forms of life is now threatened by the toxic pollutants we throw into the waters, air, and land. Many world leaders are finally coming together to confront this threat, but great changes in human habits will be required if we are to succeed in reversing the degradation of our biosphere. Each of us is being asked, both individually and as members of cities, states, and continents, to discontinue wasteful and polluting behaviors. However, if we continue to pollute our bodies internally by eating toxic foods and taking pharmaceuticals that are not absolutely necessary, it is doubtful we will ever heed the warnings of scientists to reduce our external forms of pollution. How well each one of us cares for our own internal environment is an accurate predictor of how well we will care for the external environment we all share.

So, What Do We Do Now?

Given the current state of our collective health, what options do we have for improving the strength and health of our nation and our species? The way I see it, there are only two options.

1. Do nothing. Accept the status quo. Trust political leaders who tell us they will take care of things for us. Follow passively along the current path. Remain silent in the shadows of the "authorities" who have guided us since the 1950s. Allow matters to run their course. Let things play out as they will. Continue our roles as passive Acceptors.

2. Actively Revolt against the perpetuation of the never-substantiated Diet-Cholesterol-Heart Hypothesis; educate ourselves more thoroughly in the subjects of nutrition, digestion, science, and ecology; refuse to accept health "science" reports based solely upon selected epidemiological studies that frequently are interpreted deceptively; demand that the scientific method be utilized strictly and completely, with actual honest clinical trials, before nutritional and pharmacological advice and products are subsidized and recommended to us by official organizations of the US government; purchase large amounts of vegetables and other produce as directly as possible from local organic growers; join our local food co-ops; withdraw economic support for industries and organizations that exploit every opportunity available to increase their profits while knowingly causing increased illness among all of us; exercise our rights to exercise; and use prescribed and over-the-counter medications only when truly indicated and necessary. In short, we have the capability to liberate ourselves from the bonds of colonization by disease, if—and only if—we exert ourselves thoughtfully and forcefully.

Option #1 is built upon at least one unsupportable hypothesis: if we do nothing, the status quo will be preserved. In terms of health and independence, there is no status quo. Our health and freedom—as individuals, as a national population, as a species—never stay the same.

> Every day we either become healthier or less healthy, stronger or weaker, more independent or more dependent.

Steadily, since the 1950s, the rates of obesity, diabetes, respiratory diseases, gastrointestinal diseases, neurological disease, opiate addiction, and other disabling afflictions have increased. These negative shifts have been an economic diamond mine for industries poised to exploit them, such as Big Pharma and the Medical Industrial Complex.

Alongside colonization by obesity and diet-related diseases in the US, there has been a worldwide population explosion, with greater concentrations of people living in large cities. As more of us are crammed into larger urban centers and housed more vertically, we surrender greater shares of our personal independence. Vertical cramming increases our dependence upon others to provide food, energy, water, and other necessities of life. This plays into the power-hungry palms of Big Farma, which claims the only way to feed growing urban populations is with massive amounts of cheap, highly-processed, mass-produced, grain-based foodstuffs.

As the truly scientific writer/researchers of the 21st Century have revealed, overconsumption of grain-based foodstuffs is the major reason why our rates of obesity and related chronic diseases have increased so dramatically. Obesity will only continue to increase if we continue to eat as we have been told to for more than half a century. The final logical extension of Option #1 has been immortalized in a motion picture starring Charlton Heston. In **Soylent Green,** more than 40 million people live in New York City in the year 2022. They subsist almost entirely upon wafers made from a compound of oceanic soybean mash, grains, and human remains. In this film, the Exploiters reach the summit of their dreams: totalitarian control of the human diet, health, and behavior!

As much of our health freedom as we have lost to date, we could lose even more.

Cha-Ching! Cha-Ching! Cha-Ching!

Option #2 is the American Diet Revolution, the fight to reclaim our health independence. Whether we realize it or not, this revolt began in the year 2000 when Ravnskov, Taubes, and other writer/researchers began firing bullets of the scientific method into the bloated, drug-addicted, mythical, Diet-Cholesterol-Heart Hypothesis, sugar monster. In the second decade of the 21st Century, Gundry, Davis, Perlmutter, Mullin, and many other physician/researcher/writers enlisted their hearts and minds in the fight for honesty, health, and freedom from unnecessary, preventable, chronic diseases caused by the excessive consumption of addictive and toxic foods, drugs, and other imprisoning substances. The works of these early 21st Century revolutionaries are the antithesis of the relentless prescription drug advertisements that flood television screens, the internet, and print media.

The future habitability of planet Earth depends on our collective determination as world citizens to radically change the ways we use fossil fuels and other natural resources. If we are to succeed in preserving a beautiful, natural world for future generations to enjoy, then the vast majority of us must practice honest, responsible, thoughtful, and personal stewardship of our external environment. Likewise, the future of life, liberty, and the pursuit of happiness in the United States depends greatly on our collective determination as individual American citizens to practice personal internal environmentalism. We must consider carefully the beneficial and detrimental consequences of every food and substance we ingest.

We are not a healthy people. A large majority of us are excessively fat, physically unfit, and addicted to toxic foods, drugs, and other substances. Even as the richest nation in the history of human civilization, we cannot afford adequate health care for all of our citizens because so many of us are ill and disabled. We have been colonized by chronic, preventable diseases. Our liberties are diminished because we have become unnecessarily dependent upon the powerful Exploiters who control the commodities they have led us to believe we need.

It would be wrong to declare that the chronic diseases plaguing so many Americans are due only to external factors beyond our control. There are reasons for our current states of illness other than the greed of large conglomerates. Yes, they have positioned themselves to take advantage of economic opportunities, heightened considerably, even to this day, by perpetuation of the Diet-Cholesterol-Heart Myth. However, we must acknowledge our shared responsibility, as individuals and, collectively, as a society.

We Americans, as a culture, consciously or subconsciously, have accepted an increasingly frantic pace of life. We have embraced fast cars, fast internet speeds, and fast food. We are proud of our international reputation for economic prowess and of the fact that most of us are willing to work very long hours each week and take very little vacation time each year. Gradually, we have accepted and then demanded more speed. If a computer does not boot up in two seconds, we yell "Come on!" at the monitor. If we are tired, we do not try to get more sleep, we take a stimulant to keep us going for another five hours. If we have pain, we do not slow down and give our bodies a chance to heal; instead, we start on the bottom rung of the drug ladder (non-steroidal anti-inflammatories) before climbing to opioids. We are an increasingly impatient society made up of increasingly impatient individuals. If a television news program does not deliver the information we are seeking within 30 seconds, we hit the remote to search for another channel that will. If we were not the first, we were among the first to eat meals in our cars, initially in drive-in restaurants (we eliminated the "rest" part), and soon afterward in "drive-thru" restaurants, allowing us to eat while we drive. We have become so accustomed to eating in the car that most of us don't even think about it anymore. Very few of us have paused to consider how living fast and eating on the run affect our digestion and enjoyment of food.

To be frank, we Americans have been guilty of too much passive acceptance since the end of World War II. We have accepted great economic growth and great innovations—cell phones, electric can openers, smart phones, social media, drones, and thousands of other gizmos—without really thinking through some of the consequences of such advances. We have accepted ever-increasing demands for faster and more productive performances at work and in school. We have accepted bloated cable TV bills and cheap gasoline.

We are Acceptors.

One arena of life in which we Americans have become particularly accepting is in how we expose ourselves to information. All day, nearly every day, with radios and televisions babbling in the background, or with headphones and cell phones, we encounter small bits of electronic information and ingest it as we do fast food—down the hatch while we are driving, running, or cooking. In distracted states such as these, we often don't differentiate between paid persuasion and factual reporting. We collect it all in the same bowl. We do not sufficiently question the veracity of the data we're receiving. We fail to exercise due vigilance. Without questioning its sources, we accept as factual most of the information we accumulate.

Since the 1950s we have been bombarded with the phrase "healthy whole grains." The USDA, advertisers, the American Heart Association, innumerable diet gurus, and thousands of other individuals, businesses, and organizations have spouted this three-word ditty so often that most Americans have just accepted it as one of the universal truths of life. Obediently, we have followed the advice implicit in this phrase: to increase our consumption of grains. Since 1961, we Americans have increased our intake of grain-based foodstuffs by approximately 30 percent. This dietary shift is simultaneous with increases in obesity from approximately 14 percent to 36 percent and in diabetes from less than 1 percent to more than 11 percent. Yes, these are just epidemiological statistics. They do not prove causation. However, the association is strong enough that we should at least question the truth of the decree that eating grains is healthy for human beings.

But are we being inquisitive about this assertion?

For the most part, "No!" Most of us continue in our roles as passive acceptors of information. Entities such as the American Heart Association, the American Diabetes Association, the USDA, etc. advise us to keep eating the grains, and we comply.

Just as we have accepted without question the advice that eating grains is essential for our good health, we have also accepted the bombardment of propaganda that says cholesterol is an evil substance in our bodies and that we must do everything possible to lower our total cholesterol and LDL levels. Once again, we have complied with the advice of our all-knowing authorities by decreasing the amounts of cholesterol in the foods we eat and taking statin drugs that lower the levels of LDLs in our blood (Never mind that certain LDLs are carrier molecules which deliver cholesterol to the human brain where it serves thousands of essential functions every second of our lives).

But have we questioned this advice from our "authorities?" Do we question the fact that cholesterol medications are among the most profitable commodities on the planet?

For the most part, we have remained obedient colonists; we comply without questioning. We accept.

Fortunately, growing numbers of honest researchers have published books and studies that do ask the hard questions about dietary and pharmaceutical advice that has been hammered into us since the 1950s. From these authors, we have learned how the rise of the whole-grain and cholesterol myths has been fueled by deliberate misuse of the scientific method. We have learned about the specific components of grains, especially of wheat, that cause disruption of GI function in human beings, disruption that causes hormonal imbalances, inflammation, obesity, heart disease, cancers, autoimmune diseases, and neurological diseases, to name only a few.

We must make it clear to the Exploiters—and to ourselves—that the burden of proof is now upon the shoulders of those who claim that eating grains and taking cholesterol medications are beneficial for human health. No longer can we allow Big Farma, Big Pharma, and the Medical Industrial Complex players to get away with making unsupported claims. However, because they have amassed so much money and accumulated so much control over us, they are not going to give up their profits or their power willingly. If we seek truth in our knowledge of nutrition, weight loss, and dietary health, a significant number of us must revolt, must no longer accept the dogma of the Exploiters, must initiate the fight to break the bonds of colonization by disease made possible by deceitful dietary advice and pharmaceutical exploitation. It is incumbent upon us to elevate the American Diet Revolution from the level of research to the level of rebellion. This revolt is overdue. We cannot wait any longer for it to erupt spontaneously; too many of us are too obese and too ill. If we allow the Exploiters to continue plowing along their merry paths to unlimited wealth and unchallenged power, there will be too few of us left who are healthy enough and free enough to fight back.

It is our great fortune and opportunity to be born into the first truly national democracy. Let us no longer be intimidated by money-grubbing, power-grabbing Exploiters. Because of the Constitution of the United States, we citizens still have rights, freedoms, and the means to fight back against oppression. The most powerful arms we bear are our rights: to educate ourselves; to assemble and discuss ideas and issues openly; and to wield influence via our economic choices. We have the means and the power to regain our health and freedom. We can stage our own battle of defiance, our own Boston Tea Party.

To break the bonds of colonialism by disease, we do not have to destroy the democratic system in which we live. Instead, we must make better use of the tools of peaceful liberation that our founders infused into the Declaration of Independence, into the US Constitution, and into the Bill of Rights. We owe it to our revolutionary ancestors not just to enjoy and be grateful for the rights they procured for us, but also to exercise the responsibilities they entrusted to us as citizens of the republic they created. Furthermore, we owe it to our present and future descendants to restore the liberties of good health and economic independence that have been eroded by the stealth of the Exploiters. When we are being oppressed, it is not only our right to protest, but also our duty to rebel against the forces behind that oppression. No longer can we afford to be passive Acceptors of whatever information is thrown our way. Now and always, we must be active Questioners. We must pledge to exercise our rights and duties to be vigilant, to read, to discuss, to inform ourselves, and to revolt against anyone who attempts to profit by colonizing us with disease.

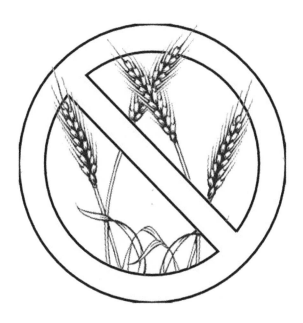

The Declaration of Health and Diet Independence

When, in the course of human events, it becomes necessary for one earnest class of people to dissolve the educational, nutritional, economic, medicinal, political, and other bands which, they discover, have been used to bind them unfairly to the whims, wills, and advantages of other exploitive individuals, groups, and organizations, then the Laws of Nature and decent Self-Respect demand that such Earnestines shall declare their intentions to alter the terms with which they shall interact with these Exploiters in the future.

We, the free citizens of the United States of America, hold these truths to be self-evident, that all of us have the rights and duties: to strive for optimal personal health; to educate ourselves thoroughly about the purity, safety, and nutritional values of the foods and drugs we choose to consume; and to avoid those foods and substances we discover can be harmful to our health and detrimental to our personal physical independence.

Furthermore, we affirm that, if and when the actions of Exploiters shall become destructive to our health and well-being, it is our responsibility as citizens to exercise our right to remove all forms of financial assistance to these oppressors and, instead, to direct our monetary support to those individuals and groups that strive to help us achieve excellent health and local community interdependence.

Furthermore, we submit respectfully that the scientific method of validating concepts of health should be applied fairly and without deception and, conversely, that when evidence is presented which documents certain groups or individuals have attempted to deceive us instead, we shall band together and boycott the purchase of any foods, drugs, or other products from such Deceivers.

In abstaining from the consumption of goods and services offered previously by deception, we pledge not to attempt to prevent the Exploiters from continuing to hawk their wares. We shall not replicate the hubris of those Exploiters who have sought to subvert the scientific method and, instead, to be recognized as omniscient. Rather, we shall support the search for truth by allowing for the open and honest execution of the scientific method.

We, therefore, citizens for nutritional honesty, health excellence, personal physical independence, and local community interdependence, do declare our intention, to the greatest extent possible, to restrict ourselves from interaction with and support of those groups and individuals who, by systematic deception, have colonized so many of us by obesity and disease. Furthermore, we do hereby declare our intentions to increase dramatically our understanding of human nutritional health, to support those in our local communities who grow, raise, and/or sell foods and nutritional products demonstrated by up-to-date science to be healthful for human beings, and in every other way, to work for truth and justice in the dissemination of nutritional information and dietary advice.

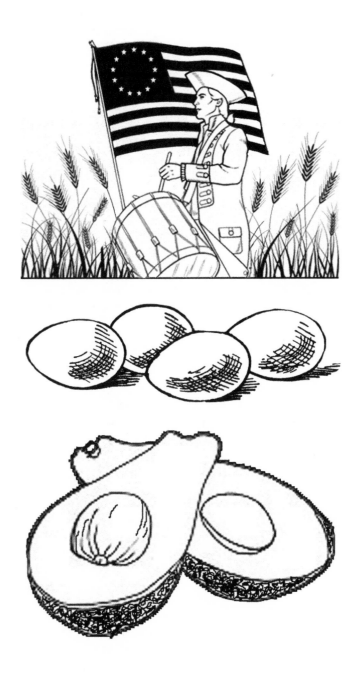

Chapter Four

American Diet Revolution
Plan of Battle

To be successful, a rebellion against the vicious cycle of oppression by disease and dependence must be based on the execution of a well-designed strategy. In this case, we do not have to use weapons of mass destruction, or even mild violence, to restore our health and freedoms. We merely must use the rights and weapons of freedom fought for by the original American Revolutionaries of 1776 and consecrated in the US Constitution and the Bill of Rights. We can restore our physical integrity and reclaim our freedoms without bloodshed. We do not have to take the Exploiters to the guillotine. Instead, we must reassert our right to lead healthy lives and enjoy our personal liberties by consigning Exploiters to their place. And their "place" is next to us—not above or dictating us—as participants in American culture.

Not all members of the Exploiters have evil intentions. Many, if not most, are actually unaware that, by taking advantage of certain opportunities in our free enterprise republic, they have helped create a large mass of colonists who have gradually become dependent on or addicted to their goods and services. In fact, many individuals who belong to the Exploiters are themselves obese and diabetic colonist victims as a consequence of consuming the very products and services they promote and profit from financially. They are both oppressors and the oppressed.

The Battlefronts

The war against colonization by obesity and disease must be fought on four environmental fronts.

1. The Personal Front

    a.   Each of us must renounce our personal role as a passive Acceptor of secondhand nutritional and dietary information and propaganda. Every one of us who is capable should become an active Self-Educator, one who reads the books and studies of scientists, healthcare providers, and other writers who are willing to submit their works to the rigorous application of the scientific method.

    b.   Each of us must establish a high degree of nutritional health within our own body by eating foods that promote excellent digestion, that supply all essential nutrients, that reverse obesity, and that nourish the microbial armies in a healthy GI tract.

    c.   If we do ingest drugs, prescribed or otherwise, we must endeavor to understand their benefits and risks, to consume only those which are truly essential to our health, and to avoid any which are unnecessary or have unacceptable side effects.

2. The Local Community Front

    a.   We all must recognize that much of our personal health freedom is based on local interdependence, that is, created directly by our interactions with the friends, neighbors, and other citizens in whose midst we dwell.

b. We must recognize and support especially the Growers in our communities, valiant individuals who work tirelessly to supply us with supremely fresh foods that nourish us and are raised in a manner that enriches the natural lands of our local external environment.

3. The National Front

a. We cannot be a strong nation if the majority of us are obese, pathologically overweight, excessively drug-dependent, or physically unfit.

b. Educating ourselves to eat more nutritiously and exercising to achieve physical fitness are essential to creating the guerilla army we need to free ourselves from the control of the Exploiters who have colonized us since the 1950s.

c. As Americans, we take pride in being leaders of the free world. During the time in which we are rebelling against industrial foodstuffs and other substances that have polluted our individual internal environments, we must strive to reverse methodologies that are polluting the air, water, land, and other elements of our external environment. We must demonstrate by example to other citizens throughout the world that a nation of enlightened people can prosper personally and collectively by cultivating the health of our internal and external environments simultaneously.

4. The Planetary Front

a. Whatever dietary decisions we make to improve our personal health—our internal environment—must include careful consideration of the impact those decisions have on the external environment of our entire planet, upon which we are all dependent for freedom and happiness. Eating fresh kiwis may be beneficial for our personal health. However, kiwis grown abroad require transoceanic transport and the combustion of substantial amounts of fossil fuel. Our personal benefits from eating imported kiwis on a regular basis may be outweighed by the degradation of our global external environment.

b. As members of the human race, we must confront the probabilities that (1) there is a limit to the number of us who can live healthfully on our planet at any one time and (2) that we may have exceeded that number already. As more and more of us are compressed into smaller geographical areas, we sacrifice proportionally more of our individual liberties, become more dependent upon the wills and acts of others, and, in effect, become increasingly colonized subjects rather than free human beings. And yet, continuing expansion of the free enterprise economic system depends on an ever-increasing population of consumers. How do we reconcile this dilemma? How do we shift from a socioeconomic philosophy in which prosperity is based primarily upon continually increasing populations of consumers clamoring for increasing quantities of goods and services to one based upon ideals of human life, such as excellent health and personal freedom? If we are concerned about the well-being of our children, grandchildren, and greatgrandchildren, and of our planet, we must face questions such as these head-on, as active self-educators, rather than evade them as passive acceptors of whatever propaganda is thrown our way.

Executing the Battle Plan

The primary goals of the American Diet Revolution are to break the bonds of colonization by disease and re-establish our collective and individual health freedoms. To accomplish these goals, we must eliminate passive acceptance of unverified dietary advice and initiate an active, but civilized, revolt against those who exploit us. This revolt *must* become widespread because, like our planet, we have reached a tipping point. Due to poor diets, so many of us are obese and diabetic now that if we delay, there will be too few of us left to fight. Today, there are just enough of us left to mount a successful revolt against oppression by food and obesity-induced diseases.

In the Bill of Rights, the founders of our republic bequeathed to us civilized weapons of self-defense by which we may liberate ourselves from any who would re-colonize us. Those weapons are the rights to read, to think, to write, to speak, to assemble, to discuss, to protest, and to influence events of commerce and governments by our economic choices. It is time to exercise these rights, to employ these weapons, to bear these arms in a well-organized militia, and to fight peacefully but forcefully for honesty and truthfulness in the battlefields of nutrition and dietary advice.

The specific, shoulder-mounted, surface-to-air weapons we can and should employ are the rights to:

1. **Educate ourselves;**
2. **Eat for Well-Being;**
3. **Economize;**
4. **Ecologize;**
5. **Exercise.**

In the following chapters, I describe specific strategies for utilizing these weapons of liberation, decolonization, and fat-mass destruction.

Chapter Five

Educating Ourselves: Armament #1

The first armament we must fire to regain our health freedom from the Exploiters is to read at least one or two works by honest, contemporary, nutritional researchers. Only through re-education can we free ourselves from the poisonous misinformation we have been subjected to since the 1950s.

The good news is that this weapon does not require a PhD. For example, most of us do not understand every detail or even much of the science behind the phenomenon of global warming. However, after reading books and articles, listening to news briefs, and viewing documentary broadcasts, most of us now have at least a rudimentary understanding of how and why accumulating concentrations of atmospheric gases—such as carbon dioxide and methane—are primary causes of our planet's increasing temperatures.

In a similar manner, to attain a basic level of understanding in the fields of nutrition, digestive health, and dietary advice, each of us needs only to read and discuss the most reliable literature available today. Such literature includes: (1) books by authors who have no ties to Big Farma or Big Pharma; (2) reports of real clinical studies conducted by researchers whose work is not underwritten and/or influenced by the economic power of the Exploiter industries; and (3) articles, documentaries, newsletters, blogs etc. by writers, producers, and others who are dedicated to discovering and sharing truthful information about the production, preparation, and consumption of the foods we eat every day and the physiological effects of those foods. These authors have documented the widespread deceit that characterized the last half of the 20th Century. Furthermore, these revolutionaries have also provided positive action steps each of us can take to free ourselves from the prisons of obesity, chronic disease, premature physical disability, and helplessness caused by the disease-inducing foods that have dominated our diets for decades.

> May the 21st Century finally be the time in which the fight for personal health freedom breaks out into a full-scale revolution against our colonization by the Exploiters!

The following is a list and brief description of eight of the most important books on diet and nutrition written and released in the 21st Century. Several of these works have already been cited in *American Diet Revolution!* and each of these books represents a significant contribution to our understanding of human health and nutrition in the 21st Century.

(1) *Wheat Belly Total Health* (2014) by William Davis, M.D. Grain-based foodstuffs constitute over 50 percent of the calories consumed by human beings. Davis identifies many of the specific components of these grass seed products—especially wheat-polluted products—that are toxic to human beings. He describes in detail why human beings experience gastrointestinal distress and tissue damage when we eat them, why even organic grains raise our blood sugar to destructively high levels, as well as why these foodstuffs cause inflammatory diseases in all the organ systems of our bodies. In short, by reading *Wheat Belly Total Health*, we gain a solid understanding of why many of the specific foods

we eat today are the predominating factors in the development of the contemporary chronic diseases that disable us prematurely. As do several of the other revolutionary physician/researcher authors, Davis includes a well-designed, gourmet-quality menu of nutritious and economical foods we can eat to replace the toxic foodstuffs that have been colonizing us by disease.

(2) *The Big Fat Surprise* (2014) by Nina Teicholz. More fluently and in more detail than any other author, Teicholz documents the origins and continuation of the dual myths that (1) fats are the main dietary cause of heart disease and (2) "heart-healthy whole grains" are instrumental to our salvation. Not content with merely reciting the summaries of the supposedly scientific studies upon which whole-grain myths were elevated to near-biblical status, Teicholz reviews much of the actual raw data upon which the Diet-Heart-Cholesterol Hypothesis was based. We see for ourselves how Ancel Keys manipulated his data to create the conclusions he wanted to be true. And we see how he and his fearful followers resorted to dirty tricks to make health claims they could not have made if they had followed truly scientific methods. These supposed scientists tricked us into believing they knew the cause of heart disease and that, if we followed their dietary advice, we would conquer the most prevalent cause of premature death in the US. By passively accepting their deceptive recommendations, we allowed ourselves to be colonized by obesity and its related chronic diseases. Teicholz's work is poignant for her descriptions of direct interviews with many of the honest researchers whose works were suppressed and ridiculed by weaker "colleagues" who gained academic prominence and reward by jumping on the Keys bandwagon. In reading *The Big Fat Surprise*, we begin to realize the extent to which selfish forces colluded and cooperated to consolidate enormous profits, prestige, and power within their ranks. As a direct result of the epidemics the Keysians helped to create, millions of Americans are disabled today by obesity and its related chronic

inflammatory diseases. Thanks to Teicholz, we now realize we cannot continue to be passive Acceptors of the Exploiter's dietary propaganda. Only by revolting actively against the misinformation they continue to spew can each of us regain our maximum potential to be healthy and physically independent.

(3) *Grain Brain* (2013) and **(4)** *Brain Maker* (2015) by David Perlmutter, M.D. We are in debt deeply to this brave physician/ researcher/author for making us aware of the neurological disease time bombs exploding in the brains of most of us today as a consequence of the toxic foods and drugs we ingest. Nothing robs a person of his or her individual health independence more completely than premature dementia. From Dr. Perlmutter, we understand that the emotional and economic costs of imprisoning so many of our fellow citizens with Alzheimer's and related neurological diseases will soon dwarf the costs of treating those of us who are incarcerated with diabetes. Like William Davis, Perlmutter not only describes the problems created by so many toxic foodstuffs, but also presents a comprehensive menu of delicious real foods to replace the highly-processed jail food we colonists have been eating since the 1950s. In addition, he offers a succinct explanation of the microbiome, the astounding environment of intestinal microorganisms that populate the GI tract of every human being and play major roles in almost all of our bodily functions.

(5) *Gut and Psychology Syndrome* (2004), Natasha Campbell-McBride, M.D. For several reasons, *Gut and Psychology Syndrome* is an essential book for us to educate ourselves about the beneficial effects of eating nutritious foods and the destructive effects of consuming foodstuffs toxic to the human GI system and, by extension, to all organ systems of our bodies. In describing the microbiome and its myriad of critical effects on human health, especially on the nervous system, Campbell-McBride predates other revolutionary writer/researchers by over a decade. In reading *Gut and Psychology Syndrome*, we begin to

understand the causes of many crippling neurological diseases that have colonized us with increasing frequency over the past few decades. Those of us with autism, ADHD, schizophrenia, dementia, and Alzheimer's Disease all have GI tracts characterized by abnormal microbial populations.

(6) ***Gut Balance Revolution*** (2015) by Gerard Mullin, M.D. From Mullin's up-to-date research and detailed descriptions, we begin to understand the intricate relationships between the quality of the food we eat, the functions of our microbiomes, and many of the physiological and pathological processes of the human body. Just like Davis, Campbell-McBride, and Perlmutter, Mullin offers a comprehensive and nutritious eating plan to achieve a healthy degree of bodily leanness. In addition, he offers guidelines for rest, exercise, and mental peace to attain higher levels of whole-body health.

(7) ***Primal Fat Burner*** (2017) by Nora Gedgaudas, CNS, NTP, BCHN. In this thoroughly referenced book, Gedgaudas broadens our understanding of how radically different our diets are today from what they were throughout most of human history. She dispels the myth that our ancestors were lumbering brutes who knew nothing about what they should eat to thrive and survive. On the contrary, we begin to see how they learned what sources of food would sustain them. In their diets, it was primarily the rich supply of saturated animal fats that fueled dramatic increases in the size of the human brain. Today, however, rather than rely upon our senses as our ancestors must have done, many of us allow external forces to determine what foods we should eat. By surrendering our independence to make food choices for ourselves, we have surrendered our health freedom as well. Gedgaudas' work is particularly distinguished by her detailed explanations of fat metabolism in human beings.

(8) ***The Plant Paradox*** (2017) by Steven R. Gundry, M.D. ***The Plant Paradox*** is a monumental contribution to our understanding of the botanical, physiological, and pathological relationships between the plants and animals we eat and our health. We learn why eating certain types of foods triggers a severe inflammatory reaction within our bodies. As an accomplished clinical researcher, as well as a practicing cardiologist and heart surgeon, Gundry details in graphic terms the pathological results when we eat foods we cannot digest easily or well. Of particular importance is his thorough examination of lectins, virtually indigestible proteins that are abundant in grains, legumes, some seeds, and many other foods. At last, we understand why we must avoid most of these foods entirely. As do Davis, Perlmutter, Campbell-McBride, and others, Gundry provides detailed menus and recipes representing his attempt to put into daily practice the nutritional principles his research supports. For instance, to reinforce his contention that we can and should restrict our intake of animal protein, he lists recipes for several vegetable-based and nut-based dishes that provide ample amounts of protein to meet our daily needs. In doing so, Gundry offers a powerful and well-reasoned alternative to a return to the "Paleo" diet in the 21st Century.

Beyond the eight essential books cited above, there are at least seven other significant works we should consider reading to achieve a more comprehensive understanding of the need for the American Diet Revolution.

1. *Good Calories, Bad Calories* by Gary Taubes
2. *Why We Get Fat* by Gary Taubes
3. *The Cholesterol Myths* by Uffe Ravnskov, M.D.
4. *Put Your Heart in Your Mouth* by Natasha Campbell-McBride, M.D.
5. *Eat Fat, Get Thin* by Mark Hyman, M.D.
6. *Smart Fats* by S. Masley, M.D. and J Bowden, Ph.D.
7. *The Case Against Sugar* by Gary Taubes

To anyone who reads even one of the 15 works cited in this chapter, it will become abundantly clear that we cannot continue to be passive Acceptors if we hope to liberate ourselves from colonization by obesity and disease at the hands of the Exploiters. She or he who goes on to read a second work will, without question, enlist as a guerilla warrior in the revolt against continued oppression by the Exploiters.

Chapter Six

Eating for Well-Being: A 21ˢᵗ Century Diet Plan

Clearly, the dietary advice drummed into us since the 1950s has not been beneficial to our health. By obediently accepting and following this advice, we became increasingly obese, diabetic, and sickly dependents of Big Farma, Big Pharma, and the Medical Industrial Complex. Now, however, we have finally begun to educate ourselves about real nutritional science and abandon the misinformation used to colonize us. But increasing our understanding of nutrition is not, by itself, sufficient to reclaim our health freedom. To realize our individual potentials for physical independence, we must wield the second armament of the American Diet Revolution: Eating for Well-Being.

So, what does Eating for Well-Being mean?

At its most basic level, Eating for Well-Being denotes selecting, preparing, and eating foods that supply our bodies with all the nutrients necessary to achieve excellent health. In addition, it means avoiding the ingestion of foodstuffs and other substances that damage any of the major organ systems of our bodies and that cause us to become obese, inflamed, and vulnerable to colonization by disease.

"Well-Being" connotes more than just the personal internal health of any one individual; it suggests that our external environment must be healthful as well. We cannot truly thrive if we live in the midst of toxic air, water, and land. Therefore, eating for well-being includes eating in a manner that is beneficial for the health of our families and friends, our neighbors and local communities, our nation, and our planet. As mentioned earlier, eating kiwis might be healthy for individual Americans. However, if the kiwis we purchase require transcontinental shipping from the South Pacific or the Mediterranean, the air pollution of their transit might outweigh the kiwis' nutritional value. An example closer to home would be eating almonds from California. While it may be very beneficial for our health, if the water requirements for raising almonds on a commercial scale are causing severe depletion of the aquifers in the American West, we must weigh carefully the consequences of consuming large quantities of this nutritious nut. In summary, Eating for Well-Being means that we have to consider all of the effects of our food choices, not only on our personal internal and external environments, but also on those of all other humans and organisms in our local, national, and global communities.

In making informed decisions about which foods we choose to purchase and eat—as well as which foods we choose not to purchase and not to eat—we are deploying a powerful socioeconomic weapon. Collectively, our food purchases have a profound impact on the economic prosperity of those of us who grow, prepare, and sell those foods. If, for instance, a sizable number of us begin to read honest contemporary nutritional research and, therefore, elect to abstain from purchasing and eating grain-based foodstuffs, there will be a drastic negative shift in national grain sales, grain transportation, grain planting, restaurant sales, bakery sales, supermarket sales, the packaging industry, and a myriad of other related enterprises.

Less swiftly, but just as surely, there will be shrinkage in the diabetes management industry, decreased obesity-related disease care, decreased hospitalizations, decreased drug sales, and so on.

Simultaneously, if our increased awareness of real nutritional research leads us to triple our purchases of vegetables, nuts, and seeds to replace the grain-based foods we eliminate from our diets, there will be a corresponding positive shift in the growing, transportation, marketing, sales, and preparation of those foods. In short, when we deploy the weapon of Eating for Well-Being, armed with the knowledge we gain from nutritional research, we unleash thunderous economic demands for honesty and justice in our food supply. In effect, we are reaching for better health by purchasing what we now know are healthier foods than the ones we have been duped into buying since the 1950s.

The following paragraphs consist of: (1) a summary of the principles of healthful eating as presented by the foremost researcher/writers of the 21st Century; (2) my recommendations of where, when, and how to buy healthy foods in a manner consistent with the well-being of our local, national, and global communities; and (3) my recommendations regarding efficient ways to purchase, prepare, eat, and enjoy the best possible foods we can obtain to realize our individual potentials for good health.

Summary of the
Principles of Eating for Well-Being

1. <u>We should not eat</u>, or limit as much as possible, foods that:
   a. are highly processed, such as lunch meats, candies, chips, soft drinks, bread, bagels, muffins, and other grain-based foodstuffs;

b. contain synthetic additives, artificial sweetening or coloring agents, chemical preservatives or flavorings, dough conditioners, monosodium glutamate, etc., etc., etc.;

c. raise our blood sugar levels rapidly, including not just sweets such as soda, juice, candy, pie, and cake, but also high glycemic grain-based foodstuffs, such as bread, crackers, and oatmeal, all of which cause the secretion of insulin, the fat-storage hormone;

d. are difficult for human beings to digest and, therefore, are not broken down easily or completely in the human GI tract;

e. foods that contain addictive compounds, such as the protein Gliadin, which is found in wheat-based foodstuffs and binds with opiate receptors in the human brain and, therefore, leads to addictive overeating;

f. cause tissue damage and inflammation of the GI tract, such as the lectin Wheat Germ Agglutinin, an indigestible protein in wheat that injures the tight junctions between cells in the small intestine, thereby leading to Leaky Gut Syndrome, autoimmune diseases, and other processes detrimental to human health;

g. have been treated with herbicides, pesticides, and artificial fertilizers, which make such foods not only toxic to humans directly, but also deficient in beneficial microorganisms essential to human health;

h. are derived from animals which have been fed or injected with synthetic compounds, unnecessary medicines, growth hormones, and/or chemically treated feeds;

i. leave us with cravings, even after we have eaten ample amounts of them;

j. cause gas, bloating, indigestion, etc.; and

k. require extensive transportation pollution to reach our local communities.

Not eating foods toxic to the human digestive system is merely the first step toward regaining our health independence. If we sincerely wish to realize our individual potentials for vibrant well-being, we must purchase and consume the most nutrient-rich and locally grown foods we can afford. Once we have discovered which types of foods offer the greatest health benefits, we must learn methods of preparing them to be delicious as well.

2. <u>We should</u> eat foods and drink fluids that:
   a. supply us with the macronutrients (fats, proteins, and carbohydrates) and micronutrients (minerals, vitamins, and phytochemicals) we need to complete all essential physiological processes of the human body;
   b. contain large and varied populations of beneficial micro-organisms to replace those our bodies eliminate every day;
   c. contain abundant amounts of fiber, soluble and insoluble, to facilitate optimal GI function;
   d. supply us with generous amounts of water in both solid foods and beverages;
   e. supply caloric energy sufficient to meet our basal metabolic needs and fuel our daily physical actions, without raising our blood sugar levels rapidly and, therefore, without triggering a massive release of insulin;
   f. are grown organically, that is, without artificial chemical treatments, with deep respect for the health of those who grow and eat them, and for the health of the environment we all share;

g. are processed as little as possible, such as fresh, raw, organically-grown vegetables, nuts, and some seeds;

h. can be purchased with as little packaging as possible, such as at farmers' markets or in the vegetable section of co-ops or health food stores;

i. do not require excessive transportation to reach us, in other words, locally raised whenever possible;

j. we enjoy eating; and, after we have eaten them, leave us feeling satisfied rather than craving more.

Principles! What Specific Foods Should We Eat?

Confronted with principles of healthy eating and long lists of the types of foods we should and should not eat, many of us have several questions and concerns, such as:

"Your list of foods to avoid includes many of the foods I have been eating for years. Now I learn I should not be eating most of them. So, what can I eat?"

"If I eliminate all the foods you tell me are detrimental to my health, I am going to starve."

"Most of the foods on the banned list are the ones that taste really good."

"How am I going to live without eating bread and bagels and muffins and pasta and crackers and juice and oatmeal? Those are some of the main things I eat every day."

Exclaimer

Those questions are absolutely fair questions, questions that must be answered if there is truly going to be an American Diet Revolution. In the next section of this chapter, we address those questions directly and in detail. Before we do, however, I offer one important reminder: do not accept what I say without doing at least *some* research yourself. Read at least one of the books listed in the last chapter. Read other books or articles on nutrition and judge for yourself if they are written with honest respect for the scientific method or, if instead, they are propaganda supported by a suspicious twisting of epidemiological data. We Americans have descended into an epidemic of obesity because we accepted advice about what we should eat without questioning the validity of that advice. Let's not make that mistake again. If we yearn to regain our freedom from colonization by obesity and its related inflammatory diseases, we must become active questioning revolutionaries. In short, I urge you to question everything written or stated by me and anyone else in the fields of nutrition and dietary advice. Not only are we what we eat, but, just as importantly, we are what we read and what we think.

Specific Foods We Should Eat
Vast amounts of Voluminous, Voluptuous Vegetables!

Virtually all contemporary nutritionists, researchers, and writers agree that, for most of us, eating a large volume of fresh, raw, cooked, and/or fermented vegetables every day is essential for good health. Whether we are vegans, ova-lactivores, or omnivores, all of us should be bona fide Vegetabletarians. Possible exceptions might be those of us who have gastrointestinal diseases, allergies, or other conditions that prevent us from digesting vegetables easily and well. Many Americans suffer from GI tract diseases and food allergies to vegetables that were originally caused by exposure to the inflammatory compounds and allergens present in grain-based foodstuffs.

For the purposes of our discussion here, the word "vegetable" is used to refer to foods that are botanically classified as vegetables (lettuce, carrots, and broccoli) and not to vegetable-like, seeded fruits (tomatoes, cucumbers, eggplant, and peppers). As Steven Gundry has revealed, the lectin proteins in the seeds and skins of such pseudo-vegetables cause inflammatory reactions in the GI tracts of humans who eat them.

"What is a vast volume of vegetables?"

"How much is a serving?"

"Why so much?"

"How can I eat that much?"

"What about the costs?"

First, we should try to eat generous amounts and varieties of dark green and brightly colored vegetables because they are very rich in the minerals, vitamins, phytochemicals and other compounds our bodies need in order to conduct a vast array of essential physiological functions in each of our organ systems every day. In most cases, these essential nutrients are highly bioavailable in vegetables, which means we can digest these foods and absorb their vital substances readily and efficiently.

Secondly, most vegetables contain large amounts of fiber and water, two substances essential for optimal human digestion but which contain virtually no absorbable calories. The combination of fiber and water makes vegetables spatially voluminous and calorically sparse; that is, they take up a lot of space in the GI tract and yet have relatively few calories. A serving of broccoli, for instance, contains about 35 calories, approximately half the calories in one slice of whole wheat bread. Within a few minutes, we can easily eat two slices of whole wheat bread (approximately 150 calories of concentrated and quickly digestible carbohydrates), cause our blood sugar levels to rise rapidly, trigger an insulin reaction, begin to store body fat, and still not feel full. However, if in the same period we try to eat four servings of broccoli—or an equivalent caloric amount of another vegetable—we will have to stop eating long before we can finish. Even if we could eat this much vegetation at one time, we would not experience an insulin reaction or cause storage of body fat because the concentration of calories from carbohydrates is lower and the process of digestion is slower in vegetables than in grain-based foodstuffs.

In short, we can eat very large quantities of most vegetables without being concerned about increasing our body fat. The amount of vegetables we can eat at any given meal is limited by the large quantities of fiber and water they contain. A great volume of vegetable matter in the GI tract stimulates nervous receptors that send impulses to the brain which, in turn, translates those signals into a feeling of fullness and a command to stop eating for a while. Thus, by gradually increasing the amount of vegetables we eat every day, we reduce our drive to fill our bellies with the addicting, fattening, diabetes-causing, pro-inflammatory, genetically-manipulated, grain-based foodstuffs that have dominated our diets for such a long time.

As an absolute minimum, we should eat five servings of fresh vegetables each day. Even the USDA—finally abandoning the sinister Food Pyramid—now urges us to eat five to seven servings of vegetables and fruits daily.

So, how much is a serving?

A serving is approximately what you are able to hold easily in the palm of one hand: a large carrot, a fistful of romaine, a couple stalks of celery. A large salad might easily contain three to five servings of vegetables.

Although eating a large salad every day might enable us to reach the minimum recommendation of the USDA, that amount is inadequate for anyone who aspires to excellent health. When we delete nutrient-poor, calorically-dense, grain-based foodstuffs from our diets, we must replace some of their calories and most of their fibrous volume with an additional three to five servings of vegetables daily. In other words, each of us should strive to become a Vegetabletarian, someone who aspires to eat seven to 10 servings of vegetables each day. At first, this may seem daunting. However, by gradually increasing the amount of vegetables we eat every day, we develop a heightened awareness of the rich variety of flavorful ways we can enjoy these nutrient-intense, calorically-sparse, voluptuous gifts of Nature. Not long afterward, we experience the joy of being leaner, healthier, and more energetic. And then, a little later in this progression, we begin to realize we have taken a significant step towards liberating ourselves from colonization.

No longer do we crave grain-based foodstuffs.

Even more than the quantity, we must consider the quality of the vegetables we eat every day. The qualities we should seek in purchasing vegetables are:

a. that they are fresh, guaranteeing their nutrients and flavors are at maximum levels;

b. that they are grown organically, and thus contain rich supplies of beneficial microorganisms and an absolute minimum of environmental toxins;

c. that they are grown locally, meaning they are very fresh, that we are supporting our local growers and local community, and that we are minimizing the earth-polluting effects of excessive transportation and packaging; and

d. that, if they cannot be purchased fresh, they are preserved in as nutritious a manner as possible, meaning they are packaged in non-toxic containers, such as in glass jars after fermentation and/or canning, or by freezing or dehydration.

The best ways to prepare and eat vegetables are:

1. **Raw**. Most vegetables can be eaten raw, as in a salad. When they are eaten raw, their native flavors and textures shine through. In addition, most of the nutrients and microorganisms are preserved and available for absorption into our GI system.

2. **Cooked lightly.** Some vegetables are broken down more easily and their nutrients absorbed more completely when they are steamed, sautéed, or cooked in soups. Oxalic acid, present in raw kale, for example, causes gastric distress for many of us. However, steaming kale for just five minutes reduces this compound dramatically, making the vegetable tastier as well as more digestible and its nutrients more easily absorbed. Other vegetables, such as Brussel sprouts, are bitter and extremely difficult to chew in their raw state.

3. **Fermented.** Vegetables, especially organically grown vegetables that have not been treated with herbicides, pesticides, fungicides, etc., have rich supplies of microorganisms living in and upon their tissues. During the process of fermentation, these microorganisms produce acids and enzymes that dramatically reduce the sugar content of a vegetable, prevent it from spoiling, and make it more digestible for humans. By eating fermented vegetables, we increase the populations of beneficial microbes in our GI tracts.

In summary, rather than a plant-based diet, we should strive to eat a **Vegetable-Based Diet**. Every day, we should eat ample amounts and varieties of vegetables that are grown organically and locally, packaged as little as possible, and prepared in all three ideal forms: raw, cooked lightly, and fermented.

A Sample List of Nutritious Vegetables

Artichokes	Aramae	Arugula	Asparagus
Baby Bok Choy	Basil	Beets	Beet greens
Bok Choy	Broccoli	Brussel sprouts	Cabbage
Carrots	Cauliflower	Celery	Chives
Collards	Cilantro	Dandelion greens	Escarole
Endive	Fennel	Garlic	Green Beans
Kale	Kelp	Kohlrabi	Mizuna
Mushrooms	Okra	Onions	Parsnips
Parsley	Radishes	Scallions	Shallots
Sea vegetables	Seaweed	Spinach	Leeks
Sweet potatoes	Swiss chard	Turnips	Turnip greens
Wakame	Watercress	Yams	Kimchi

The vegetables named above constitute only an exemplary list, not an encyclopedic one. As you shop for produce at farmers' markets, food co-ops, and health food stores, as well as in progressively-managed supermarkets, you will encounter many vegetables not found on this list. Half of the thrill of being a Vegetabletarian is trying new vegetables. So be brave! Go wild! Try a new vegetable every week!

Ample Amounts of Fabulous Fats!

One of the tragic consequences of the dietary deception of Americans in the second half of the 20th Century is that even today, we have dramatically reduced the amount of healthy fats in our diets. Real nutritional scientists then, as well as physicians who kept themselves up-to-date by reading nutritional research, knew this was a mistake, knew that consuming generous amounts of fats was essential for good health. However, their shouts for rational science were drowned out by others clamoring to jump on for a free ride on the Diet-Cholesterol-Heart Hypothesis trolley car.

The following outline presents a partial list of many of the types of healthful fats each one of us should consider for our personal diet. As with vegetables, we must choose our fats based upon quality first and, only secondarily, with regard to quantity. Unlike vegetables, but like protein foods, such a list also needs to be differentiated to meet the needs of those of who are vegan vegetabletarians, ova-lactivore vegetabletarians, or omnivorous vegetabletarians. Therefore, fats of non-animal origin are listed first and are appropriate for everyone, followed by those derived from eggs and milk, and then those directly from animal tissue. In addition, fats on this list are categorized according to their types: saturated, monounsaturated, polyunsaturated, etc. However, please keep in mind that this is an oversimplification. In most foods, fats are of mixed types, some saturated, some monounsaturated, some polyunsaturated. The foods listed are categorized by their most abundant class of fat for simplicity's sake.

A. Saturated Fats—from local, organic sources whenever possible
  1. Saturated fats—Vegan Vegetabletarians
     a. Coconut, coconut oil, coconut butter, coconut manna—all organic. Perhaps the most versatile of all fats, coconut is delicious when eaten raw right out of the shell. Coconut oil is superb for cooking, even at moderately high temperatures, as well as in smoothies and homemade nut butters. Coconut butter and manna can be used as natural low-sugar toppings, as flavorings, or eaten right out of the jar.
     b. Red Palm oil, sustainably raised, for cooking, smoothies
     c. Cacao—raw nibs or powder, sustainable and organic
     d. nuts, seeds, nut/seed oils: macadamia, walnut, sesame

      e. avocado oil

  2. Saturated fats—Ova-lactivore Vegetabletarians

      a. Eggs—from local, pasture-raised chickens

      b. Clarified butter (ghee) from local, pasture-raised cows, goats, or sheep

      c. Sour cream, whole-milk yogurt, kefir, or raw-milk cheese from local, pasture-raised cows, goats, or sheep

  3. Saturated fats—Omnivore Vegetabletarians

      a. Meat fat from local, pasture-raised cows and lambs

      b. Meat fat from locally raised, organically fed pigs (e.g. bacon)

B. Monounsaturated Fats

  1. Monounsaturated—Vegan/Ova-lactivore

      a. Olive Oil—extra virgin, first cold-pressed, organic

  2. Monounsaturated—Omnivore

      a. Lard and/or Tallow from locally pastured cows and pigs

C. Polyunsaturated Fats

  1. Polyunsaturated—Vegan/Ova-lactivore

      a. Brazil nuts, pecans, almonds, walnuts, hazelnuts, macadamia nuts, etc.—raw and organic

      b. Flax, hemp, and sesame seeds, all organic and raw

      c. Avocados—organic

  2. Polyunsaturated—Omnivore

      a. Fish and fish oil—wild-caught, sustainable species, fresh-water, salt- water; shellfish from clean ocean areas

      b. Poultry fat—from local, pasture-raised birds

In the list above, note that for each type of fat, qualitative descriptions are included, such as, "local," "organic," "pasture-raised," or "wild-caught." To achieve optimal health, it is essential that we eliminate as many potential toxins from our foods as possible. This is true particularly of animal fats. Most of the poisons, toxins, drugs, and other substances animals encounter in the air, water, and soil—as well as in their foods and injections—are stored in their fat cells. Therefore, for those of us who choose to eat animal-based foods, it would be foolish to eliminate toxins from plant-based foods but continue to ingest them from impure animal fats. Therefore, we should endeavor to purchase and consume animal foods that have been created as purely as possible. A steer raised on GMO corn and soybeans, treated with synthetic growth stimulants, injected relentlessly with antibiotics, and forced to stand constantly in a crowded muddy feedlot will have dozens of volatile toxins in its body fat. By comparison, if its twin grazed on unpolluted grass in open pasture and did not receive either antibiotics or growth stimulants, it would have relatively few toxins in its body fat.

As I mentioned earlier, a significant percentage of the calories in our diets should come from fats. They are a superb source for the energy our bodies require to execute all the processes of life. However, many foods that are predominantly fat have little or no fiber and water and thus, per calorie, have relatively little volume compared to vegetables. For this reason, my recommendation is that we should eat only moderate quantities of fats; they are so dense calorically that we do not need to eat large volumes of them to fulfill our nutritional needs. For example, a tablespoon or two of olive oil and half a dozen Brazil nuts sprinkled on a salad may provide more calories than are contained in all the voluminous voluptuous vegetables in that salad.

Moderate Amounts of the Purest Proteins Possible!

We human beings require adequate amounts of dietary protein nearly every day of our lives to meet our structural and functional needs. By including high-quality sources of protein in our diets, we supply the building blocks necessary to repair and replace the cells and tissues that are constantly breaking down in our bodies. How much protein each of us needs is highly variable. To meet her metabolic and growth needs, a teenage athlete needs more protein in her diet than her grandmother does. However, the qualities of the protein foods we eat are more important than the quantity. By far, we are much healthier if we eat modest quantities of high-quality protein foods rather than large quantities of poor-quality proteins. A major purpose of this section is to define and explain what distinguishes high-quality protein foods from low-quality protein foods.

The first quality we must consider is whether a specific protein food comes directly from plants or if it comes from animals. How well humans can digest and utilize protein from each of these sources varies significantly. In general, the proteins in foods from animals are far more concentrated and can be utilized more readily in the human body than the proteins in most plant foods.

Proteins are composed of chains of specific amino acids, many of which must be available during the digestive process to enable humans to absorb and utilize such protein efficiently. Although our bodies can synthesize many amino acids internally, there are at least eight essential amino acids we must get directly from the foods and other substances we ingest. Most plant protein foods are deficient in at least one essential amino acid, thus limiting how much protein we can assimilate and use from these foods if they are eaten in isolation. By contrast, most animal foods contain more complete supplies of essential amino acids. Therefore, in general, the proteins in animal foods can be broken down and utilized more efficiently than protein in plant foods.

The human body does have ways to compensate for the relatively incomplete amino acid profile of most plant foods when they are compared to animal foods. If plant foods and animal foods are eaten at the same meal—or even during the same day—the human digestive system can use some of the essential amino acids from the animal sources to assimilate the plant proteins more completely. For the same reason, during the course of every day, we should eat several different types of plant foods. When we eat a wide variety of plant-based foods every day, their differing concentrations of amino acids complement each other. This means more of the protein from each plant food is available for use in a person's body than if he or she had eaten only one or two types of plant foods on that day.

(Count this as one more reason to eat a great variety of vegetables every day.)

The second and most important quality of protein foods we elect to purchase and eat is their purity. As with vegetables and fats, if we are striving to reach our individual potentials for well-being, we must select and consume protein foods that are as pure as possible. Pure plant protein foods are grown organically, without the use of pesticides, herbicides, chemical growth stimulants, or any other toxic substances or methods. Pure animal foods come from animals that have not been injected with drugs and growth hormones and that have been raised in environments as close as possible to their native outdoor grasslands or woodlands. Even food products from "organically fed" animals are not healthful for humans if their feed was from sources high in lectins, such as corn or soybeans. In addition, we should avoid eating foods from animals confined in cages stacked high in industrial factory buildings or penned knee-deep in muddy feedlots. Whether we consume toxins directly from plants or indirectly from the animals that eat such polluted plants, the results are largely the same. We become repositories for the toxic chemicals in those chemically-treated foods. Although the human digestive processes can eliminate some of the toxins in polluted protein foods, many of the industrial substances remain in our bodies indefinitely, even permanently. Whether they remain in our bodies for hours, days, or for the rest of our lives, these toxins are major causes of inflammation, obesity, and chronic, preventable, disease processes.

As with all our food purchases, we should strive to buy protein foods from our local growers and "ranchers," local food co-ops, local health food stores, local butchers, etc. People we know personally are the ones we can place the greatest trust in to offer us the purest foods possible.

Specific Protein Foods Classified by Source

We human beings fall into three classes of eaters, based on the sources of the foods we choose to consume:

1. **Vegans,** who eat only foods from plant sources;
2. **Ova-lactivores,** who do not eat animal flesh but do eat eggs and/or dairy foods;
3. **Omnivores,** who eat foods from all sources, including animal flesh.

Each of us makes deeply personal choices regarding the sources of our foods. No attempt is made here to convince a reader to alter his or her choices. Instead, in the following lists, protein foods are presented separated by source. Vegan protein foods are listed first because they are available for all three types of eaters. Protein foods for ova-lactivores are listed second, followed by protein foods for omnivores.

Protein foods for Vegans—from Local Growers whenever possible

1. Raw Organic Nuts:
    a. Almonds
    b. Brazil Nuts (good source of complementary amino acids)
    c. Pistachios
    d. Pecans
    e. Macadamias
2. Raw Organic Seeds:
    a. Hemp

    b. Flax

    c. Walnuts

    d. Sesame (good source of complementary amino acids)

3. Organic Vegetable and Fruit protein sources:

    a. Mushrooms

    b. Avocadoes

4. Organic Legumes (in very small quantities due to lectin proteins):

    a. Only fermented organic soy: tempeh, natto, miso

    b. Beans cooked in a pressure cooker to reduce lectins

5. Vegan Organic Protein Powders, especially Hemp Protein

6. Organic Nut Milks, especially Almond Protein Milk

7. Organic Brewer's Yeast and Nutritional Yeast

Protein Foods for Ova-lactivores—from Local Growers whenever possible

1. All protein foods listed above for Vegans—except legumes— plus

2. Eggs from Pasture-raised chickens, ducks, etc.

3. Dairy Products from Pasture-raised and Grass-fed cows, goats, and sheep

    a. Whole-milk yogurt

    b. Whole-milk kefir

    c. Raw Whole-milk cheeses

    d. Whey, goat/cow/sheep protein powders for shakes and smoothies

Protein Foods for Omnivores—from Local Growers whenever possible

1. All protein foods listed above for Vegans and Ova-lactivores, except legumes

2. Beef, Lamb, Pork, and Chicken from Pasture-raised animals

3. Wild-caught, sustainable, low-on-the-food-chain fish from pristine waters, especially:
   a. Sardines
   b. Herring
   c. Anchovies
4. Bone Broth from the bones and connective tissues of Pasture-raised, Local, Grass-fed animals
5. Shellfish from certifiably clean waters

At first, the lists above may appear to be very limited. Notable for their absence are all protein sources from grain-based foodstuffs. As discussed earlier in this book, the lectin proteins in grain-based foodstuffs are extremely difficult for almost all human beings to digest. Such foods often cause or contribute to leaky-gut syndrome, intestinal inflammation, auto-immune diseases, food addictions, and a myriad of other debilitating disease processes. In addition, modern, grain-based proteins are housed with concentrated, high-glycemic carbohydrates that elevate human blood sugar levels rapidly and for sustained periods of time, factors which inevitably lead to frequent and intense insulin responses, obesity, diabetes, and, eventually, dementia and other preventable and disabling diseases.

Liberal Amounts of Luscious Libations!

One of our first nutritional goals each day should be to make sure we consume a generous quantity of fluids, especially pure water. By drinking a variety of liquids every day, we can also provide ourselves with many essential nutrients. Therefore, although the list below begins with water, it also includes several other elixirs of well-being.

A. Drink moderate amounts of pure or purified water throughout the day. One of the most common dietary missteps we can take is failing to consume enough clean water each day to meet our metabolic needs. We are frequently victims of the hectic pace of contemporary life. Because we focus so intently on the seemingly important external demands of the day, we ignore internal signals that we are thirsty. When we finally realize we are parched, we are already somewhat dehydrated, meaning we may have compromised the functions of our kidneys and other organs. One of the simplest ways to prevent dehydration is to keep water at hand all day long. As soon as you wake in the morning, drink a cup of water before you drink or eat anything else. Keep a bottle or two of water at your desk, in your lunch box, and in your car. If you feel hungry between meals, try drinking a cup of water before eating or drinking anything else. You might be thirsty rather than hungry. As with other foods and drinks in our diets, we must seek the purest sources of water possible to reduce the risk of contaminating our bodies with toxic substances. In the case of water, even if your municipal water supply is clean when it leaves the water works, it may pick up contaminants as it careens through miles of piping before emerging from the kitchen faucet. At a minimum, use a countertop filtration pitcher to ferret out as many toxins as possible. Under-the-sink and whole-house filters are also available and affordable. Alternatively, purchase reverse-osmosis filtered water at your local food co-op or health food store.

B. **Drink a cup of bone broth daily. If you are a vegan, substitute a cup of vegetable broth.** Both are rich sources of minerals that we may not be able to absorb in adequate amounts from the foods we eat. Bone broth, one of the most nutrient-dense foods available, has the added advantage of being a rich source of protein. By now it should be obvious that we must purchase broth that comes from local, pasture-raised animals. To economize, we should buy bones and make broth ourselves. Vegetable broths should be derived from organic sources.

C. **Eat vegetable soups made with bone broth and pure water.** This is a grand slam home run. In just two cups of soup, we can satisfy significant amounts of our daily needs for protein, pure water, minerals, vitamins, and fiber.

4. Drink one or two cups of blissful beverages every day. Fruit juices are hyper-sweet fatteners, not healthful drinks. If your goal is to **increase** your body fat substantially—or if you merely want to retain all your current body fat—drink orange, apple, or grape juice and you will attain both objectives. Instead of gulping down high-glycemic juices, grain-sweetened sodas, or overpriced sports soft drinks, we can enjoy delicious, satisfying, and healthful beverages, such as the examples below:

   i. Coffee and tea, caffeinated or decaffeinated, are both rich sources of anti-oxidants. In addition, the fiber in coffee is an excellent prebiotic delicacy feasted upon with gusto by the beneficial flora in the human gut. If you enjoy rich, smooth, creaminess, whip either beverage in a blender with organic coconut oil and/or pasture-raised ghee, both of which are excellent sources of saturated fats.

   ii. Green Tea is rich in anti-oxidants and available in dozens of delectable flavors.

   iii. Kombucha, fermented green tea, is loaded with probiotics to replenish the armies of microorganisms that camp out in the GI tract and are essential for normal function in all organ systems of the human body.

   iv. Herbal teas are superb, non-caffeinated, non-caloric, midday or after-dinner beverages to satisfy the lingering desire for something sweet and flavorful. There are literally hundreds of different flavors of herbal teas, some of which are reputed to impart glorious health benefits to those who drink them.

E. **Nutritional shakes and smoothies, Vegan or Ova-lactarian.** We think of these first as rich sources of protein, fiber, and vast amounts of nutrients, which they are. However, they also contain generous amounts of water and, thus, count toward satisfying our daily fluid needs.

F. **Concentrated Vegetable Drinks.** One of the easiest ways for all of us who are Vegetabletarians to meet some of our needs for phytonutrients and water every day is to purchase concentrated organic vegetable powders and mix a teaspoon or two in 8 to 12 ounces of cold clean water. In seconds, we have a refreshing power drink that is low in sugar but abundant in micronutrients that would be extremely difficult to gather from local vegetables alone.

Small Quantities of Low-Sugar Fruits!

Like most vegetables, which are nutritional powerhouses for human beings, many fruits are rich reservoirs of essential nutrients. Some foods we think of as vegetables, such as avocadoes, are actually low-sugar, high-fiber fruits. Many brightly colored fruits—such as strawberries, blueberries, and cherries—contain generous amounts of microscopic polyphenols that neutralize the corrosive actions of free radicals, rogue compounds, that invade and degrade all organ systems of the human body. On the other hand, relative to vegetables, most fruits have a high sugar content. In addition, the seeds of many fruits have high concentrations of lectins, which we must avoid. Therefore, we must be very careful about the types and quantities of fruits we consume.

Just as we do with vegetables, fats, and proteins, we should endeavor to purchase fruits that are grown organically and locally. Fruits grown with industrial fertilizers, herbicides, fungicides, and pesticides retain residuals of those chemicals that cannot be removed by washing or even peeling away the skins. Additionally, those industrial toxins destroy most or all the beneficial microbes living in and on such fruits, which diminishes their nutritional value even further. We need to take in billions of these beneficent microorganisms from the foods we eat every day in order to replenish those our bodies eliminate. In addition to their substantial nutritional value, low-sugar fruits serve other important roles in our diets, such as satisfying our desire for flavor and sweetness.

Okay, enough fruit theory. So, what specific types of fruit should we eat, how much should we eat, and when should we eat them?

Low-Sugar Fruits, organically grown if possible, up to 1cup/day

1. Avocadoes
2. Blueberries (especially wild blueberries)
3. Raspberries
4. Cranberries
5. Blackberries
6. Pomegranate kernals

Clearly, this is a very limited list and is not adequate to satisfy either our nutritional needs or our desires for flavor, sweetness, and variety from the dozens of delectable fruits available to us. On the other hand, we can't ignore the fact that most fruits have high concentrations of fructose (fruit sugar). The answer to this dilemma is to eat fruits with moderate concentrations of sugar at strategic times and in controlled quantities. In other words, we should consider fruits in a special way in order to enjoy their sweet flavors and benefit from their nutrients, while preventing them from causing blood sugar surges, obesity, and related diseases.

First, let's consider fruits as the amazing masterpieces of nature they are. In a natural, unprocessed, raw state, their flavor is more exciting than virtually any other food type. Right off the vine or the stem, without any treatment, most ripe fruits are sweet and luscious. They are a gift to humankind, as well as to our animal friends. Therefore, fruits must be revered and respected, treasured, eaten slowly, and appreciated. When we eat fruits slowly, we savor every mouthful. By eating them with the concentrated attention they deserve, we can experience them fully without eating excessively large quantities.

One way to eat fruits with honor and respect is as a special snack between meals, rather than as part of a full meal where they have to share the glory with other foods. When we eat them alone, the sugar in the fruit is not added to the sugar content of other foods, lowering the risk that we will cause a massive insulin reaction. In addition, the fiber content of many fruits is enough to slow down digestive breakdown, further inhibiting blood sugar spikes.

One other special attribute of fruits must be noted. They help humans bond. That is, they are an ideal food to be shared. If we give half of a fruit to a friend or loved one, we are eating only half the sugar, but the sweetness we taste from the shared experience far exceeds that which we would have tasted had we eaten the whole fruit alone. The following list is a sample of fruits with moderate sugar levels.

Moderate-sugar fruits: eaten between meals, in small amounts (<1/2 cup)

1. Small diameter (< 2 ½") tart apple (Granny Smith), organic
2. Small juice oranges (whole, not juiced) organic
3. Strawberries, organic
4. Grapefruit, organic
5. Small organic pears
6. Organic kiwis
7. Organic cherries

8. Organic peaches, plums, nectarines
9. Strained tomatoes and tomato sauce

Some of the nutritional researchers, writers, and physicians of today advise against eating any fruits such as these because of their fructose content. However, I side with other authors who feel that we do need the occasional pleasure of a little sweetness in our diets and, if we eat fresh, ripe, local, organic fruits in very small quantities, then the fiber, antioxidants, and other nutrients they contain will offset some of the negative consequences of fructose.

Straining tomatoes removes the seeds and skins of the fruit, thus reducing their toxic lectins. We can use strained tomatoes to add flavor to many of our favorite cooked dishes, such as cabbasagna (more on that later).

We can also consider eating relatively high-sugar fruits, such as bananas, mangoes, papayas, and plantains, when they are green, before their sugar content becomes high. If we incorporate these green gems into smoothies, they add a great deal of texture, prebiotic food for our microbiota, and other nutritional treasures to our blender concoctions. In addition, some organic, dried fruits—such as figs and dates—contain many important nutrients. Most of us can enjoy these occasionally as desserts. Again, they taste especially sweet when we share them with friends and loved ones.

Superb Snacks

Almost all of us experience times between meals when we feel hungry but have no nutritious food readily available to eat. In some such instances, we are dehydrated rather than hungry, and a tall glass of pure water cures our "hunger" pangs. On the other hand, there are times when we are truly hungry and could use a small quantity of food to bridge the gap until our next full meal. For moments such as these, it is wise to have a small stash of healthy snack foods close at hand. We've already talked about a few examples of such foods:

- Organic berries, cherries, and other low-sugar fruits
- Organic raw coconut flakes
- Organic raw walnuts, almonds, etc.

If we combine members from all three of those groups in a small jar or bag, we have a homemade trail mix that can travel with us almost everywhere we go, always ready to save us from fat-fast-food joints and convenience-store food facsimiles. Whether fresh from the shell or dried and flaked, coconut is a particularly spectacular snack food because it has a satisfying sweet taste and it requires extensive chewing, which slows us down considerably as we eat it.

Another nutritious snack food is the tigernut, which is not really a nut, but rather, a small (about the size of a chickpea), very fibrous, sweet-tasting, root vegetable. Because they are so chewy, it is advisable to soak tigernuts in water overnight before attempting to eat them. Tigernuts contain a significant quantity of resistant starch, a carbohydrate that does not break down rapidly, does not raise human blood sugar levels quickly, and provides food for the microbial armies in the GI tract.

We've also talked about some other types of healthy foods that function well during snack attacks. Bone broth, green and herbal teas, and concentrated vegetable drinks are just a few examples of between-meal boosters that can be transported easily in a travel mug and be ready for deployment at the first sign of hunger. These all have the added benefit of supplying us with water, which we all need generous quantities of throughout the day.

Savory Spices and Heavenly Herbs!

There is almost universal agreement among leading contemporary nutritional writers and researchers that our diets should include several varieties of fresh and dried spices (from the berries, bark, roots, and fruits of vegetation) and herbs (from the leaves, flowers, and fleshy stems of plants).

First, when used well, spices and herbs infuse our foods with a stimulating array of exciting flavors and aromas. By seasoning our foods with these magical mini-vegetables, we free ourselves from the twin tyrannies of sugar and salt, our addictions to which are exploited on a massive scale by the barons of boring industrial foodstuffs. Herbs and spices reawaken our senses of smell and taste. If we yearn to liberate ourselves from the fat-fast-food of the Exploiters, we must redevelop our willingness to try new flavors.

Secondly, and just as importantly, many spices and herbs are storehouses of medicinal substances that are immensely beneficial to all who consume them. Just by sprinkling tiny amounts on our solid foods, or adding them to soups, broths, and teas, or taking them as supplements, we enhance our immune system capabilities, stimulate our metabolisms, and provide our bodies with natural phytochemicals essential for optimal human function.

As with every food and liquid substance we consume, we must seek the purest forms of spices and herbs we can find. Many of these tiny food treasures can be purchased fresh and organically grown at farmers' markets, natural food co-ops, or health food markets. Co-ops and health food stores also carry dozens of dried herbs and spices in ecological and economical bulk bins, allowing us to buy them in limited quantities and without excessive packaging.

The list of herbs and spices we can enjoy is very long. An effective way to discover which ones appeal most to your personal senses of taste and smell is to try a new one every one or two weeks. Start with some basic ones, such as the ones in the following list.

- Basil
- Cinnamon
- Garlic
- Ginger
- Oregano
- Rosemary
- Turmeric

There are different health benefits attributed to each of these herbs and spices. Although many of these benefits have yet to be confirmed by rigorous scientific testing, all these micro-vegetables have cultural histories dating back thousands of years. Therefore, at the very least, spices and herbs provide our lives with a wonderful variety of sensory experiences.

Delectable, But Not Detrimental, After-Dinner Desserts (and Other Artful Dodges)

Once or twice a day, nearly all of us yearn to eat something delicious and maybe a little sweet. This is especially true after the evening meal, when we might feel like kicking back and treating ourselves to a tasty reward for all we have accomplished throughout the day. Therefore, a great challenge looms:

"How can I satisfy my desire for something luscious without raising my blood sugar to a point where it triggers a massive insulin reaction?"

One high-glycemic dessert after dinner—a piece of pumpkin pie, for instance—can convert what would have been a body-fat-burning day into a body-fat-storing day. However, we can proactively conquer this challenge by consuming foods or beverages that have great taste but do not raise blood our sugar levels.

Creating new habits like this demands secret weaponry; enter…

... Six Nighttime Weapons of Fat-Mass Destruction

1. Eat foods with flavors that overwhelm a sweet tooth

Often, when we eat foods with strong flavors, our yearning for sweet foods diminishes or disappears entirely. This is particularly true of foods with a powerful but delightful sour taste. For instance, two heaping tablespoons of well-bred sauerkraut after dinner not only provides one's GI tract with reinforcements for the microbial national guard, but also stimulates our taste buds with an invigorating sensation so strong that any previous desire for sweetness all but vanishes. If having sauerkraut after the main course is a little too much, try a cup of kombucha, fermented green tea with the effervescence of seltzer and, in most flavors, miniscule amounts of sugar. In addition to being a thirst quencher, kombucha is loaded with friendly microbial critters.

2. Drink a cup of herbal tea

A quick scan of the "Tea" section in a health food co-op, store, or supermarket reveals that there are literally hundreds of different herbal tea flavors from which to choose. If you try one new flavor every month, you will develop a repertoire of many favorites in a relatively short period of time.

In the evening, a sweet-tasting, non-caloric, herbal tea (such as licorice flavor) will often satisfy one's desire for something sweet and does so without adding any sugar to our diet. Alternatively, an herbal tea with strong flavor (peppermint or lemon zinger) makes such a powerful impression on our sense of taste that we forget that only a few minutes before we were yearning for something sweet. In between these two alternatives are less distinctive herbal teas (for example, chamomile) that can be sweetened, if desired, with an organically grown, non-caloric sweetener such as stevia.

3. Eat foods high in fat, fiber, and taste but with little or no sugar

- Organic Unrefined Coconut Butter (Manna)

- Raw Organic Pecan Butter
- Raw Organic Almond Butter
- Raw Organic Walnut Butter
- Raw Macadamia Nut Butter
- Organic Coconut Flakes

No bread, crackers, or other fattening grain-based foodstuffs are necessary. Nut butters are delicious when spooned directly from the jar into your mouth. When these luscious healthy fats have been pre-chilled in the refrigerator, their rich flavors and creamy textures are sensational, reminiscent of ice cream, but without the sugar. Because nut butters have thick and slightly sticky consistencies, it is advisable to have a glass of water close at hand, in case things get to be a little too gummy in your mouth.

Whether you make your own nut butters in a super blender at home or you purchase them at your local co-op or health food store, it is best if the nuts are raw. The roasting process utilized in most commercial nut-butter productions alters the oils of the nuts and destroys many of their beneficial nutritional properties.

Another fabulous and delicious food replete with beneficial fat and fiber but low in sugar is high-cacao-content chocolate. When cacao butter is removed from the cacao bean, the result is cacao powder, which, in turn, is used to make chocolate. The higher the percentage of cacao in a chocolate bar, the lower the sugar content, the more intense the chocolate flavor, and the more concentrated are the beneficial nutritional components, such as fiber and antioxidants. Therefore, when we are selecting an organic chocolate bar for health and pleasure, we should look for a super-dark one with at least 80 percent cacao content, preferably 85 or 90 percent. With this concentration of cacao, the amount of sugar should be very low, perhaps only two grams in a serving. That is, for one-quarter of a very large bar. If you allow only one small square at time to melt on your tongue, it is likely that your craving for chocolate will be satisfied with only four or five pieces, which together constitute less than one-quarter of a bar.

4. Floss and Brush Your Teeth Right After Dinner

If flamboyant flavors, herbal teas, and high-fat, high-fiber, or even high-cacao foods cannot quell your after-dinner or late-night urges for sweetness, it is time to bring out the heavy artillery. Before you grab a slice of this or box of that or a dish of something sugary, try brushing and flossing your teeth thoroughly. The taste of herbal toothpaste will dim your desire for grain-based gooey goodies. Also, the prospect of having to brush and floss your teeth again in a few hours provides a strong incentive to avoid eating again before you go to sleep.

5. Take a Walk

One of the most effective methods to keep our post-prandial blood sugar levels from rising too fast and too high—and thereby triggering a massive insulin response—is to take a 20-minute walk soon after eating. Even if deployment of the first four weapons fails to prevent you from overindulging in a fattening, grain-based dessert, taking a walk can mitigate the damage. A brisk stroll soon after dinner reduces the level your blood sugar will rise to relative to the level it would have risen had you merely continued to sit on your duff. Once we are ambling, we are reminded, once again, that a brief walk is also a fabulous stimulant for creative thinking or great conversation with a loved one.

6. Go to Sleep!

We cannot eat if we are asleep. The longer we stay up at night, the greater the opportunity to eat more than we should later than we should. The more fatigued we become, the more tempted we are to try eating food for the energy to stay awake. These are just a few of the reasons why we should try to go to sleep early in the evening (9 or 10

P.M.) rather than later (11 P.M., midnight, or beyond). While we are sleeping, our bodies go into caloric deficit, harvesting stored body fat, helping us reach optimal human health.

* * *

This completes my summary of many specific foods that we should try to eat frequently to achieve excellent health. They comprise the "What" of the American Diet Revolution. In the next chapter, we will place those foods onto specific menus, demonstrating how they can be precisely integrated into our busy daily lives. However, before we move on, we must address several other questions about the foods we've just discussed:

How should we prepare them?

How much of them should we eat?

Where should we purchase them?

Where should we eat them?

When should we eat them?

Why should we eat them?

How, How Much, Where, When, and Why Should We Eat for Well-Being?

How should we prepare the foods of the American Diet Revolution?

The value of nutritious foods to our health is greatly dependent on how those foods are prepared. We can efficiently assimilate the nutrients of many non-grain, plant-based foods when those foods are eaten raw. By contrast, the nutrients of other plant foods—such as kale, broccoli, and spinach—are more bioavailable when such foods are cooked lightly. However, our ability to assimilate the vitamins, minerals, phytonutrients, and fiber of virtually all foods is significantly diminished by overcooking, either from excessive cooking duration, high cooking temperatures, or microwaves.

The short message: we should purchase fresh foods frequently and prepare them promptly and carefully. Below is a list of seven convenient ways we can prepare high-quality foods for maximum nutritional value and enjoyment in our far-too-hectic contemporary world:

1. as salads—the quintessential way to integrate varieties of raw vegetables;
2. as soups and broths—complete protein, water, and vegetable meals;
3. by sautéing—add fat, flavor, and finesse to vegetables and meat;
4. by steaming briefly—to make vegetables just tender enough;
5. as shakes/smoothies—drink-anywhere nutritional powerhouses;
6. as trail mixes—travel-everywhere bolts of fiber, fat, and protein; and
7. by fermentation—to replenish our essential allies in the GI tract.

Each of these methods of preparation has advantages that make it a delicious, practical, and economical way to consume wholesome foods in a manner that preserves their vital nutrients. In the sample menus in the next chapter, we will see how all these favorable forms of food fit easily into our daily lives.

How Much Nutritious Food Should We Eat for Well-Being?

In addition to considering how we should prepare the nurturing foods we purchase, we should consider how much of those foods we eat.

Should we measure precise amounts of each food we eat or beverage we drink?

Should we count calories?

Grams of Carbohydrates? Grams of Fat? Sugar? Fiber? Protein?

To answer questions such as those, we have to first consider the qualities of the foods we eat and only secondarily the quantities.

Why?

If we select and eat the types of foods from which we can readily assimilate the nutrients our bodies need, our hormone levels will be more favorably balanced, and we'll feel satisfied. Foods of high quality are, to a great extent, self-regulating. They do not cause our blood sugar levels to rise rapidly. Therefore, they do not trigger an explosive secretion of insulin and a concurrent suppression of leptin and glucagon—hormones that signal when we have eaten enough and enable us to burn stored body fat.

In other words, the quality of the food we eat helps us to control the quantities of the foods we eat by modulating the hormones that control hunger. Conversely, if we eat foods of poor quality, the resulting hormonal imbalances compel us to eat greater quantities of food than our bodies need.

So, what are the characteristics of high-quality foods?

They are: (1) grown organically and locally; (2) fresh; (3) free of pesticides, herbicides, preservatives, artificial flavors and colors, and other synthetic chemicals; (4) easily digestible; (5) minimally processed; and (6) not addictive. Foods of high quality also: provide rich supplies of healthy fats, fiber, and proteins; contain generous amounts of beneficial microorganisms for the GI tract; and do not cause unhealthy spikes in blood sugar.

Earlier in this chapter, we looked at the qualities of many specific foods that are beneficial to our health, as well as the negative attributes of other foods detrimental to human well-being. Beyond the foods and food types which have been named explicitly, however, there are two alternative ways to judge if other foods are beneficial or detrimental to our health.

If we are judging the nutritional value of foods that are not pre-packaged (such as vegetables, fruits, nuts, or seeds in open bins, or meats in a butcher case), we may read the display signs or speak directly with the farmer-marketeer, store attendant, or butcher where such foods are offered. If the signs or vendor tell us the vegetables are organically raised or the meats are from pasture-raised animals, we have reasonable assurance that these foods possess some or many of the nutritional qualities we're seeking. We might also be assured that these foods are free of artificially administered chemicals that might drive us to eat greater quantities of them than we should.

For instance, meats impregnated with the salt-and-sugar taste of monosodium glutamate or originating from animals raised on growth hormones might compel us to eat larger quantities than we would have eaten if the meat from those animals had not been so treated. Nuts or seeds that have been roasted and salted will drive us to eat them in much larger quantities than if we eat them raw and unsalted.

If we are considering purchasing pre-packaged foods, we have another source of information from which to make a decision: the food label. By federal law, the label on most packaged foods must include a list of ingredients and a table called "Nutritional Facts," the latter of which lists the total weight of the product and the weight of a single serving, as well as specific numbers of grams and calories of fat, carbohydrates, and proteins, respectively. Consider the label below of Mystery Food #1.

The "Ingredients" section on the label of this food—omitted above to disguise its identity—contains only one listing: "organic dried coconut flakes," one of the superb snacks previously cited. In the "Nutrition Facts" section of this label, "Total Fat" sits at the top of the list of macronutrients (proteins, carbohydrates, and fats). It sits there because the Food and Drug Administration (FDA), from which this labeling

Nutrition Facts

13 servings per container

Serving size   **3 Tbsp (15g)**

Amount Per Serving

Calories   110

	% Daily Value*
Total Fat 10g	**13%**
Saturated Fat 9g	**45%**
Trans Fat 0g	
Cholesterol 0mg	**0%**
Sodium 5mg	**0%**
Total Carbohydrate 4g	**1%**
Dietary Fiber 2g	**7%**
Total Sugars 0g	
Includes 0g Added Sugars	**0%**
Protein 1g	**2%**

*The % Daily Value (DV) tells you how much a nutrient in a serving of food contributes to a daily diet. 2,000 calories a day is used for general nutrition advice.

originated, wanted consumers to be fearful of getting too much fat in their diets. Placing "Fat" at the top, with "Saturated Fat" on the line immediately below, was intended to discourage people from buying foods with significant amounts of fat. Now that many revolutionary writers and researchers of the 21st Century have shown how it is essential to include generous amounts of purely sourced fat—including saturated fat—in our diets, the prominent position of "Fat" at the top of the FDA food label is convenient for exactly the opposite reason of its originally intended purpose. Rather than shunning fat, we should shop for foods with labels indicating generous amounts of high-quality fats derived from organic and/or pasture-raised sources. Thus, the FDA label makes it easy to see that this is a food with the types of high-quality fat we should be seeking in many of the foods we purchase.

Other important points to note in the label above are that the grams of "Dietary Fiber" under the "Total Carbohydrate" heading are relatively high (half of the carbohydrate total) and that the grams of "Total Sugars" are almost non-existent.

In summary, by considering just three or four factors on this label, we can hypothesize that this is a food which will be self-regulating, a food which we will not eat in large quantities. The high fat content suggests that this food will be satisfying to our palates. The relatively high fiber content of this food will contribute to our feeling of fullness and initiate signals to stop eating. And, because it contains negligible amounts of sugar, this food will not cause a sudden spike in our blood sugar levels, will not initiate a fat-storing insulin reaction, and will not create a desperate urge to eat huge quantities.

Nutrition Facts

6 servings per container

Serving size   4 ounces (119g)

Amount Per Serving

Calories   350

	% Daily Value*
Total Fat 0.5g	**1%**
Saturated Fat 0g	**0%**
Trans Fat 0g	
Cholesterol 0mg	**0%**
Sodium 370mg	**16%**
Total Carbohydrate 85g	**31%**
Dietary Fiber 3g	**11%**
Total Sugars 48g	
Includes 48g Added Sugars	**96%**
Protein 5g	**10%**

Not a significant source of vitamin D, calcium, iron, and potassium

*The % Daily Value (DV) tells you how much a nutrient in a serving of food contributes to a daily diet. 2,000 calories a day is used for general nutrition advice.

Now, consider the information on the label for Mystery Food #2.

The nutritional profile of this food contrasts significantly with coconut flakes. In the "Ingredients" section of this label, the first two items listed are "organic whole wheat pastry flour" and "organic cane sugar." This label represents the nutritional profile of one organic pumpkin muffin in a package of six, just the right type of whole grain, low-fat food recommended by the USDA food pyramid of 1992. In the "Nutritional Facts" panel, we notice right away that the amount of fat in this monster muffin is tiny. No fat, no weight gain, right? Of course, we are stunned by the amount of sugar. Even though this muffin is 100 percent organic, taking two bites of it guarantees an acute insulin secretion/fat storage response. In the 20th Century, we were duped into focusing primarily on "Calories" and "Total Fat" grams and were told not to worry much about the rest of the numbers on the Nutritional Facts label. This is a quintessential example of how labeling was used in the last century to lure unquestioning Americans into the colonies of obesity, diabetes, heart disease, etc.

Where Should We Eat Nutritious Food?

While purchasing and preparing supremely nutritious foods are two very important factors in eating for well-being, where we eat those foods also has a significant impact on our physical and mental health. In general, we should make a determined effort to eat in a place that is attractive, comfortable, and sufficiently quiet to daydream if we are alone or to carry on a relaxed conversation if we are with companions. We should not eat solid food while driving, watching television, sitting in front of a computer, in bed, or even reading. Activities such as these distract us from truly smelling, tasting, chewing, swallowing, and enjoying the foods we are eating. We are inclined to gulp and swallow such foods before we have chewed them well, which disrupts normal digestion. Before we realize it, the foods we thought we were eating are gone and our brain tells us we still need more food pleasure. Therefore, we are driven to seek more food. A frequent result of this frantic scenario is that we wolf down another super-fattening, grain-based foodstuff. In the end, we have eaten much more food than we would have eaten if we had been sitting quietly at a table and savoring every morsel.

In addition to eating while distracted, oftentimes we eat in loud and hectic spaces, such as the food courts in malls, which do not provide a positive environment for optimal digestion. Even if we choose to eat the best possible foods, much of their potential value to our health is lost in chaotic surroundings that interfere with our ability to digest food well.

If your life is so hectic that you cannot possibly find time and space to eat slowly in a peaceful place and, therefore, you must eat some of your meals "on the go" or "on the job," take those "meals" in liquid forms. For instance, while you are typing you can sip a shake or broth from a large travel mug that can keep the contents cold or hot for hours. At the least, you won't be swallowing solid food that should be chewed first. However, no matter how frantic the pace of your life, make a determined effort to eat at least one peaceful, undistracted meal every day. You might find such a meal to be so pleasurable that you decide to rearrange your schedule to eat like this more often!

Realistically, most of us choose to indulge occasionally in a non-nutritious, fattening food—ice cream, for instance. Unless you have a severe food allergy, diabetes, or another health condition that excludes such an indulgence, it may be okay for you to have a "food goof" once a week. If you eat plentiful amounts of highly nutritious food every day, your digestive system and your armies of beneficial microorganisms should be able to break down and eliminate some of the excess sugars from an occasional dessert. However, again, where you eat makes a difference. If you want to cut down on your splurges with ice cream, for example, make it a personal policy to avoid purchasing half-gallons or even quarts to bring home. Instead of slurping down a quart of ice cream in front of the TV, go into the best ice cream parlor in your area, sit down, take your time, and enjoy yourself there. If you long for ice cream and there is no "sit-down" parlor in your locale, try a pint of a non-sugar, coconut milk alternative (such as SoDelicious blue label), sit in the most peaceful place in your home, and allow every spoonful to melt slowly in your mouth.

When Should We Eat Nutritious Food?

The first and most obvious answer to this question is: "When we are hungry." This answer, however, is not as useful as it appears. The physical sensation of hunger is driven by complex physiological interactions. For instance, after we eat a high-glycemic, grain-based breakfast (such as a bowl of oatmeal with milk and a banana and a glass of orange juice), our blood sugar levels skyrocket. In response, the hormone insulin is released to transport excess blood glucose into our cells and to the liver, thus lowering our blood sugar concentration back to stable levels, at least temporarily. Frequently, a few hours after an insulin reaction to elevated blood glucose, our blood sugar levels may drop, stimulating the desire for more food. Even though we have eaten a substantial amount of food only a short time before, we feel as though we are hungry which, in turn, causes us to seek another sugar fix, such as a bagel. In short, the qualities of the foods we eat, not just the quantities, have profound effects on our sense of hunger. Therefore, we cannot rely upon hunger alone to determine the best times to eat for optimal health.

Beyond the sense of hunger, another way to guide the times in which to eat for well-being is by showing respect for the human digestive system. The sensitivity and efficiency of the GI tract varies greatly from individual to individual. The Keysians and Big Grain Profiteers of the last half of the 20th Century ignored human digestion almost entirely and did not express concern about our personal sensitivities to particular types of foods or the times we ate. In brainwashing unsuspecting Americans with the unsupported Diet-Cholesterol-Heart Hypothesis, their primary goals were to gain as much prestige, power, and profit as possible for themselves and for their supporters. We mere mortals do, in fact, need to consider the physiology of our digestive systems to manage the times we eat if we wish to realize our potential for good health. Four examples follow.

During the day, allow 3 to 4 hours between each meal. This period allows your digestive system enough time to complete most of the upper GI processes of breaking down foods and absorbing their nutrients before you send down another meal. Abstaining from eating more food for four hours is much easier if the meal you have just eaten is not laden with addictive, grain-based foodstuffs. A breakfast consisting of a bagel with cream cheese, a banana, and a glass of orange juice will launch your blood sugar levels into the stratosphere, followed soon by low blood sugar, and then, an hour or two later, by the urge to get another quick carbohydrate fix. Meanwhile, the protein gliadin is binding with the opiate receptors in your brain. However, if instead you were to have an omelet with generous amounts of vegetables, a side dish of greens with olive oil and spices, and a cup of coffee or tea, you would feel fortified and satisfied for hours.

Often, we have the urge to eat food when, in reality, we are dehydrated. If you get the urge to eat between meals, your first reaction should be to **slowly drink a delightful glass of water**, spiked with lemon or lime if you prefer. If that still is insufficient to satisfy your hunger until the next meal, try eating a handful of berries or nuts, or two tablespoons of sauerkraut, any of which can tide you over until the next whole meal.

Endeavor to stop eating three or more hours before you retire to sleep for the night. We should allow time for the upper GI tract to complete most of its tasks before we place ourselves in a recumbent position. Many people experience gastric reflux if they lie down too soon after eating.

Try to go 12 hours or more between the last bite of your last meal one day and the first bite of your first meal the next day. In essence, three hours of food abstinence after dinner plus 7 or 8 hours of sleep constitute a mini-fast, a time in which your body can complete many of its essential systemic processes without the distraction of digesting food eaten recently. When you rise in the morning, drink a large glass of water before you consider eating or drinking anything else. Usually this tactic will allow you to prolong the overnight fast for another hour or two. Obviously, the mini-fast technique may not be advisable for someone who is diabetic, hypoglycemic, or afflicted with another condition dictating that he or she should not go so long between meals. As always, your personal health status and the advice of your personal physician take precedence over general guidelines such as the ones presented here.

Why Should We Eat for Well-Being?

Eating for Well-Being is a strategic fight for our personal health independence, the American Diet Revolution. If we eat cheap, mass-produced, industrialized, grain-based foodstuffs, we become helplessly obese, prematurely-disabled inmates in prisons of disease controlled by the Wardens of Exploitation. On the other hand, by educating ourselves thoroughly about the foods we choose to eat, we begin to regain both our personal health and our personal independence.

By eating well, we are not only caring for ourselves individually, but are simultaneously inspiring our fellow citizens. Each of us who advocates eating nutritious foods for well-being becomes a teacher, a revolutionary soldier, a leader who shows others by example how to revolt against the Exploiters, those who profit most when we are sickened with lifelong, diet-mediated diseases.

* * *

We've now completed a survey of: what specific foods and types of foods we should eat to achieve excellent health; how we should purchase and prepare them; and where, when, and why we should eat for well-being. Before launching ourselves into specific recipes and daily menus—which reveal how great foods can fit easily into our modern lives—it is useful to review the foods we must avoid. Eating foods that supply the nutrients our bodies need is essential. However, just as importantly, we must avoid the toxic rat bait that has dominated the American diet frontier since the 1950s.

Sample Categories of Specific Foods We Must Avoid Eating to Regain Our Health Independence

Highly processed foods

Soda, juice, chips, cookies, muffins, crackers, pastries, bread, bagels, oatmeal, candy, lunch meats, hot dogs and other commercially raised meats and animal products, sugars, and artificial sweeteners are just a very few obvious examples of highly processed foods. Less obvious examples are granola, rice, and all wheat-based foods. All foods made from grass seeds (wheat, corn, rice, oats, etc.) are highly-processed foods. They must be thrashed, pulverized, and baked before we can even attempt to eat them. And even then, we cannot digest many of their intrinsic components, such as wheat germ agglutinin. Let's be blunt here: the more processed foods are, the more money goes to the processors and the less nutrition is received by the consumer.

Foods that raise blood sugar concentrations to high levels, rapidly, repeatedly, and for prolonged periods

Since the 1980s, physiologists have been able to measure how eating different types of foods affects human blood sugar levels. First, they established the Glycemic Index, in which blood samples are drawn from a person during the first two hours after he or she eats 50-gram servings of various types of foods. These measurements are then compared to the level to which a 50-gram serving of pure glucose would raise one's blood sugar level which, for sake of comparison, is assigned a Glycemic Index number of 100. The result is a comparative number, relative to glucose, for each food. For instance, 72 is the Glycemic Index of whole wheat bread. A typical slice of bread—even organic whole wheat or multi-grain bread—will raise a human's blood sugar level as high and as rapidly as a tablespoon of sugar. In simple terms, eating bread raises your blood sugar rapidly, causing an acute insulin response and beginning the cascade to fat weight gain, diabetes, etc.

Because we do not usually eat most foods in 50-gram packages, physiologists developed the concept of the Glycemic Load, a measurement for the effect on our blood sugar levels when we eat realistic quantities of foods. For instance, they might measure the glycemic load of a breakfast consisting of a bowl of oatmeal with raisins or banana slices, a piece of toast, and a glass of orange juice. By now, you should be well aware that a meal like that will trigger a massive insulin secretion and lead directly to fat storage and obesity, and often to diabetes, cardiovascular disease, cancer, dementia, and even more massive profits for the Exploiters.

With the possible exception of commercially prepared meats, all the processed foods from the first category rapidly raise our blood sugar concentrations to high levels and are major causes of the obesity and diabetes epidemics. Among those foods, wheat (even organic whole wheat), corn, and oats have especially high glycemic indexes and high glycemic loads. Those who continue to recite mindlessly the deceitful phrase "whole healthy grains" are ignoring serious pathological effects that occur when human beings attempt to eat these grass seeds.

Foods that are difficult to digest.

Once again, all the highly processed foods in the first category are examples of industrial commodities that generate enormous profits for Big Farma, Big Pharma, and the Medical Industrial Complex, but which do not promote optimal human digestion. Among these, foodstuffs manufactured from modern wheat are preeminent because they contain specific proteins—such as wheat germ agglutinin—that are not broken down completely in the human digestive system.

These incompletely digested proteins putrefy and lead to damage in the tight junctions between cells lining the small intestine, resulting in leaky gut syndrome, seepage of abnormal protein compounds into the bloodstream, autoimmune diseases, and a wide variety of other serious health disorders. Therefore, if you desire to reach your individual potential for excellent health:

Abstain from grains, the fossil fuels of the American diet.

As evidenced by the flatulence they cause, legumes are another class of foods that are difficult for most people to digest. If after eating beans you feel bloated or gassy, it is a clear indication that their lectins are causing GI distress. Among legumes, soybean foods can be especially difficult to digest. Possible exceptions, however, are three fermented organic soy foods: tempeh, natto, and miso. Vegans, whose choices for nutritious proteins are very limited, often elect to eat small servings of legumes if their lectin content has been reduced by treatment in a pressure cooker.

Like grain-based foodstuffs, beans are high in phytates, which inhibit our ability to assimilate zinc and iron. Therefore, ova-lactivores and omnivores, who have a wide variety of protein foods from which to choose, should avoid beans completely.

Foods that contain synthetic additives

Sodium benzoate, high fructose corn syrup, artificial flavorings, artificial colors, aspartame, mono- and di-glycerides, nitrites, and nitrates are merely a few among hundreds of chemical agents added to commercial foods solely to increase profits with no regard for the health consequences for those who eat them. The simplest way to avoid being a victim of these toxins is by refusing to purchase any food with a list of ingredients that includes words you cannot pronounce. The best way to avoid these substances is to buy single-source foods in their native states from local growers whom you trust. When you buy a head of cabbage from a local organic farm stand or farmers' market, you can be reasonably assured that your food is not laced with chemicals added to prolong shelf life, disguise color, attract your eye, suck in your sweet tooth, or, in some other deceitful way, manipulate you into buying it.

Foods grown with the use of pesticides, herbicides, fungicides, artificial fertilizers, etc. In other words, "Conventionally Grown" foods.

Residuals from industrial farming chemicals always remain in the foods on which they are applied. In addition, administration of these drugs to plants greatly diminishes or destroys entirely the populations of beneficial bacteria that would otherwise be present in these foods and that, if they were present, would be of benefit to our digestive systems. In the modern global economy, the most powerful way each of us can revolt against chemical farming is by refusing to purchase any food that is not grown organically. Economic boycott is a potent revolutionary weapon.

Foods from animals that have been fed or injected with growth hormones, antibiotics or other drugs, or that have been raised on feed grown with "Conventional" pesticides, herbicides, fungicides, and fertilizers, etc.

When we eat foods such as meat, eggs, or dairy products derived from chemically-treated animals, we are ingesting the same drugs and hormones into our own bodies. Indiscriminate exposure to powerful chemicals is never a recipe for excellent health.

80 percent of the antibiotics administered in the USA are to animals.

Foods that are addictive.

When we eat foodstuffs that rapidly raise blood sugar concentrations, only an hour or two later, when our blood sugar levels have plummeted, we begin searching for more food to supply energy. Among blood-sugar-raising foodstuffs, products made from wheat are among the worst because of gliadin, an intrinsic protein of modern wheat that can cross the blood-brain barrier and bind with opiate receptors. Once we introduce addictive proteins such as gliadin into our bodies, we forfeit a great deal of our personal health independence. By abstaining from grain-based foodstuffs, especially wheat products, we are revolting personally against our own colonization by food. When we encourage those we meet, know, and love to educate themselves about what is in the foods we eat, we are contributing to a society-wide revolution against colonization by obesity and disease.

* * *

In summary, there are several characteristics in common among the most colonizing of the food products we Americans have been eating since the 1950s. The vast majority of these products are mass-produced, chemically grown and treated, highly-processed, pro-inflammatory, highly acidic, allergenic, addictive, autoimmune-disease-causing, grain-based foodstuffs. Those of us who succumb to the enticements of cheaply-made industrial food are surrendering our independence and moving toward a state of complete colonization by disease and disability. If you want a horrifying glimpse of what such a world might look like in the future, I suggest you watch the movie **Soylent Green**.

Chapter Seven

Eating Well in Everyday Practice: Armament #2

Specific Menus and Recipes

The purpose of this chapter is to present representative examples of daily food diaries for three distinct types of American Diet Revolutionaries: Vegan, Ova-lactivore, and Omnivore. As meals are described for each of these three types of patriots, the specific recipes for some of their foods, dishes, and/or meals are also presented. However, this is <u>not</u> a comprehensive diet plan. Several of the revolutionary writers of the 21st Century—for example, Davis, Perlmutter, Campbell-McBride, Mullin, Gundry, Hyman, Gedgaudas, Masley, and Bowden—have published complete dietary plans, often with assistance from accomplished chefs. As we educate ourselves by reading their works, we can follow their detailed programs to the best of our individual abilities. Those of us with patience and well-developed kitchen skills will be able to carry out their plans with precision.

In contrast to the works of the writers cited above, the primary purpose of *American Diet Revolution!* is to help as many of my fellow citizens as possible to understand: (1) how and why harmful and deceptive dietary advice has caused a high percentage of us to lose our physical health independence, and (2) that powerful individuals and groups who profit by our colonization have tremendous financial incentives to convince us we should continue our current dietary practices. I am merely summarizing the accomplishments of my 21st Century revolutionary predecessors, demonstrating how vital it is that we read their works, and—if you are convinced they are correct—urging you to follow their dietary advice rather than the deceptive 20th Century recommendations of the Exploiters.

In further contrast to the previous revolutionary writers of the 21st Century, I do not have the patience, knowledge, or skills to prepare elaborate meals or culinary masterpieces in the kitchen. Like many American citizens, I work too many hours and am involved in too many other outside activities to be able to devote much time to preparing nutritious foods. Although I enjoy making sauerkraut at home, my current schedule usually only allows me to go to my local food co-op and purchase organic kraut made by a small local producer. Therefore, most of the meals or foods described in the following sample menus and recipes can be prepared in 10 minutes or less.

For those readers who, like me, have yet to gain mastery over the tempo of our crazy contemporary world, I hope this practical approach allows you to eat nutritious foods at every single meal. For those readers who have the skill and patience to prepare their meals in a more relaxed manner, may the eating plans of Davis, Perlmutter, Hyman, Gundry, et al provide you with a great variety of more elaborate, nutritious, and delicious dishes from which to choose.

* * *

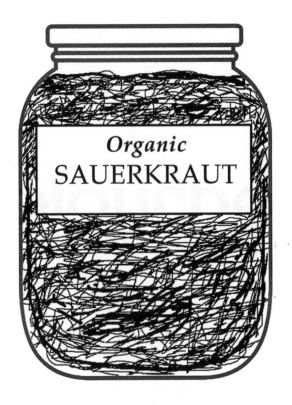

I. **Breakfast** (always with organic vegetables, nuts, seeds, and/or fruits)

    A. **Vegan Vegetabletarian**

        1. **Scrambled Tempeh with sautéed vegetables**

            a. Sauté crumbled organic tempeh in coconut oil; add scallions, garlic, kale, celery and spices.

            b. Enjoy with 8 ounces of organic kombucha.

        2. **Grain-free, Nut and Seed, Blueberry, Almond Crunchola**

            a. In a bowl mix ground flax seeds, sesame seeds, walnuts, pecans, etc. with coconut flakes, blueberries, cinnamon.

            b. Pour in 4 to 8 ounces of almond protein milk; spoon and chew.

    B. **Ova-lactivore Vegetabletarian**

        1. Vegetable Medley Omelet cooked in pasture-raised butter

      a. Cook chopped onions, spinach, chard, mushrooms for 5 minutes.

      b. Fold veggies into pastured eggs and cheese; cook 3-5 minutes.

      c. Enjoy with green tea and side dish of sauerkraut.

2. Pasture-raised, whole-milk goat yogurt and friends

      a. Into 3 to 6 ounces of plain goat yogurt, stir in almonds, pistachios, blackberries or raspberries, etc.

      b. Add a spoonful of pecan butter or tiny bit of stevia.

      c. Enjoy with a cold, green vegetable drink.

C. Omnivore Vegetabletarian

1. Pasture-raised turkey bacon, eggs sunny-side-up, pals

      a. Cook bacon in pastured butter on low heat; when brown,

      b. slide bacon to the side of the pan, cover with spinach and spices; simmer while eggs are cooking sunny side "up".

2. Breakfast Smoothie in a mug (Prepared the night before)

      a. In a blender with 8-12 ounces of water, add flax and/or sesame seeds, pastured whey protein powder, brewer's or nutritional yeast, cacao powder, cinnamon, coconut oil; blend for one minute.

      b. Add 8 ounces of coconut milk or almond milk, salad greens, any vegetables or berries you have, ice cubes, and blend until smooth and creamy. Pour into your travel mug and sip at work.

II. Mid-morning Snacks

A. Vegan Vegetabletarian

1. ½ of an avocado or small apple, orange, or pear
2. Raw trail mix: pecans, brazil nuts, walnuts, blueberries

3. Sea vegetable broth

B. Ova-lactivore Vegetabletarian

1. Boiled egg
2. Handful of cherries

C. Omnivore Vegetabletarian

1. Bone broth-1-2 cups
2. Carrot/celery sticks

D. Any and All Vegetabletarians

1. Pint of Pure Water
2. Cup of herbal tea

III. Lunch (from organic and/or pasture-raised sources)

A. Vegan Vegetabletarian

1. **Large leafy green and brightly colored vegetable salad** with raw almonds or brazil nuts, olive oil, apple cider vinegar, spices
2. **Miso and vegetable soup** with celery, onions, garlic, etc.

B. Ova-lactivore Vegetabletarian

1. **Broccoli, scallion, and strained tomato quiche** with cheddar cheese and an almond flour crust
2. **Fermented red cabbage, goat cheese, and walnuts**

C. Omnivore Vegetabletarian

1. **Dandelion greens, radish, carrot, red cabbage, and scallion salad** with sardines, squeezed lemon, spices, and macadamia nut oil dressing
2. **Leftover, pasture-raised chicken drumstick** with a side salad of fermented beets, greens, and carrots

IV. Mid-afternoon Snacks (organic and/or pasture-raised sources)

A. Vegan Vegetabletarian

1. Bowl of organic blueberries/strawberries

2.   One cup of seaweed broth
B.   Ova-lactivore Vegetabletarian
   1.   Glass of pastured, whole-milk kefir plus handful of walnuts
   2.   2-3 ounces of raw-milk pastured cheese with all-flaxseed crackers
C.   Omnivore Vegetabletarian
   1.   Afternoon Nutritional Smoothie: Blend regular or decaf coffee, whey protein or hemp powder, cacao powder, flax seeds, coconut butter, cinnamon, and ice cubes into a cool smooth froth.
   2.   One mug of pasture-raised bone broth
   3.   Pint of pure water

V.   Dinner (organic and/or pasture-raised sources)
  A.   Vegan Vegetabletarian
    4.   **#1. Vegetable and Nutty Casserole**: Sauté cauliflower, leeks, garlic scapes, mushrooms, sesame seeds, blackberries, pecans, and spices in coconut oil for ten minutes; then bake for one hour at 325°.
    5.   **#2. Coconut milk, cream of mushroom soup.** Sauté mushrooms in coconut oil with onions, carrots, and spices. Cool, add coconut milk, mix in a blender. Pour into a sauce pan. Cook on low heat 10 minutes.
    6.   **#3. Sauté a large Portabello "burger," with onions, garlic and spices in macadamia nut oil;** serve on bed of endive, chives, scallions.
  B.   Ova-lactivore Vegetabletarian
    7.   **#1. Egg Drop Onion Soup**. Heat onion soup and then drop in three eggs per person. Cook until whites are white but yolks are still soft. Add cheese and spices to suit your tastes.

8. **#2. Large leafy green and brightly colored vegetable salad.** Into a large bowl of your favorite raw veggies, mix raw pistachios, cheese, hard-boiled eggs, sour cream, chives, vinegar, olive oil and spices.

C. **Omnivore Vegetabletarian**

9. **#1. Cabbasagna.** Modify traditional lasagna. Use strained tomatoes and substitute red cabbage leaves for lasagna noodles (see pp. 136-7).

10. **#2. Small, pasture-raised pork chops.** Sauté chops and onions in butter. Smother with sauerkraut and fresh raspberries.

VI. **After-Dinner Desserts** (organic and/or pasture-raised sources)

A. **Vegan Vegetabletarian**

1. Small dish of chilled walnut, pecan, or almond butter
2. Coconut butter or coconut flakes
3. Fresh blackberries, blueberries, cherries, or strawberries
4. Herbal tea

B. **Ova-lactivore and Omnivore Vegetabletarians**

1. 2-3 ounces of lactose-free sour cream from pastured-raised goats, sheep, or cows
2. 1-2 ounces of 85 percent or more cacao content chocolate bar

* * *

One of the most effective methods for monitoring the relative healthfulness of our diets is to keep a one-week nutritional diary of everything we eat during that time. When we are forced to write down all the foods we consume during a seven-day period, most of us are quite surprised. The process of recording the foods we eat can be very instructive in improving our diets, decreasing our body fat, and liberating ourselves from the clutches of those who would like to profit from our colonization by obesity and disease.

To demonstrate how I attempt to apply the principles of Eating for Well-Being to my own life, I've included one of my own one-week nutritional diaries. Always, I strive to eat organic, pasture-raised, and locally grown foods.

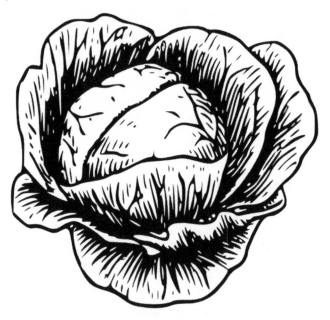

Strength for Life® One-week Nutritional Diary

Name: J Arnould

Dates: 01/06 to 01/13

Day One: 01/06

6:00 am: Water, kraut, supplements*

Day Two: 01/07

6:00 am: Water, kraut, supplements*

Breakfast: 9:00 a.m.

Vegetables: Raw Carrot

Fats: Coconut oil in smoothie

Protein: Protein Smoothie

Other: Coffee / 2 Tbsp raw walnuts

Breakfast: 9:00 a.m.

Vegetables: Carrots / celery

Fats: coconut oil in smoothie

Protein: Protein Smoothie

Other: Green Matcha Tea/ sauerkraut

Snack: 1/2 Orange, water

Snack: 1/2 pear, water

Lunch: 1:00 p.m.

Vegetables: Salad in a jar

Fats: Egg yolks, olive oil in salad

Protein: 3 soft-boiled eggs,

Other: Pistachios in salad

Lunch: 1:30 p.m.

Vegetables: Cabbage/Veg in Soup

Fats: Chicken fat in soup

Protein: Chicken/Bone-broth soup

Other: Carrots, onion, celery in soup

Snack: 1 cup Bone broth

Snack: Trail Mix

Dinner: 7:00 p.m.

Vegetables: Raw Vegetable Salad

Fats: Olive oil on salad w/ walnuts

Protein: Chicken/walnuts on salad

Other: 8 oz. Kombucha

3 oz. Pastured sour cream

Dinner: 6:30 p.m.

Vegetables: Steamed broccoli, onions

Fats: Butter/Fat on Pork Chop

Protein: Pork chop baked w/onions

Other: 8 oz. Kombucha

2oz./88% Cacao choc. bar

Day Three: 01/08

6:00 am: Water, kraut, supplements*

Breakfast: 9:00 a.m.

Vegetable: Veggies in smoothie

Fats: Coconut oil in smoothie

Protein: Whey protein smoothie

Other: Coffee/2 Tbsp sauerkraut

Snack: Bone broth

Lunch: 12:15 p.m.

Vegetables: Large salad/asparagus

Fats: Olive oil / butter(veg)

Protein: Roast beef/mushrooms

Other: 1 cup of vegetable soup

Snack: Trail mix, water

Dinner: 8:00 p.m.

Vegetables: Celery/onion sauté

Fats: Butter in Turkey/veg sauté

Protein: Ground turkey

Other: 6 oz. Red wine

3 oz. Pastured sour cream

Day Four: 01/09

6:00 am: Water, kraut, supplements*

Breakfast: 9:00 a.m.

Vegetables: 3 oz. Fermented beets

Fats: Egg Yolks/ brazil nuts

Protein: 2 Jumbo eggs, 2 brazil nuts

Other: 4 oz. kefir

Snack: Trail mix, water

Lunch: 12:00 p.m.

Vegetables: Vegs in Turkey soup

Fats: 1/2 Avocado

Protein: Turkey/mushrooms in soup

Other: Black Tea

Snack: Bone broth

Dinner: 8:00 p.m.

Vegetables: Large Vegetable Salad

Fats: Goat Cheese and olives

Protein: Chicken drumstick, cheese

Other: 6 oz. red wine

2oz./88% Cacao choc. bar

2 Tbsp of Almond Butter

Day Five: 01/10

6:00 am: Water, kraut, supplements*

Breakfast: 9:00 a.m.

Vegs: Green veg mix in smoothie

Fats: Coconut oil in smoothie

Protein: Hemp protein smoothie

Other: Coffee/ fermented beets

Snack: Trail mix

Lunch: 1:00 p.m.

Vegetables: Salad in a jar

Fats: Olive oil

Protein: 3 oz. of Sardines

Other: Sauerkraut

Snack: Bone broth

Dinner: 8:00 p.m.

Vegetables: Steamed Swiss chard

Fats: Butter on chard

Protein: Chicken breast sautéed

Other: 8 oz of kombucha

2 oz. sour cream w/flax seeds

Day Six: 01/11

6:00 am: Water, kraut, supplements*

Breakfast: 9:00 a.m.

Vegs: Green Veg mix in smoothie

Fats: Coconut oil in smoothie

Protein: Whey Protein Smoothie

Other: Coffee/ 2 Tbsp sauerkraut

Snack: Small apple, water

Lunch: 1:00 p.m.

Vegetables: Salad in a jar

Fats: Egg yolks, olive oil on salad

Protein: 3 Jumbo eggs/soft-boiled

Other:

Snack: Trail Mix, water

Dinner: 8:00 p.m.

Vegetables: Large Veg Salad

Fats: Olive oil, pecans, walnuts

Protein: Leftover chicken breast

Other: 6 oz. red wine

2 Tbsp of Pecan Butter

Day Seven: 01/12

6:00 am: Water, kraut, supplements*

Breakfast: 10 a.m.
Vegetables: Mixed veg omelet
Fats: Olive oil/butter
Protein: 3 egg omelet, turkey sausage
Other: Coffee, cream, salad greens

Snack: Tiger nuts

Lunch: 2:00 p.m.
Vegetables: Fermented beets, 3 oz.
Fats: Whole-milk yogurt, flax seeds
Protein: Yogurt, flax, walnuts
Other: Kombucha, 8 oz.

Snack: Bone broth

Dinner: 7:00 p.m.

Vegetables: Large Veg. salad
Fats: Cheese, sour cream dressing
Protein: Grilled chicken

Overview of Current Weekly Diet

Strengths: Vegs@ most meals

Raw X; Fermented X; Cooked X
Clean proteins X
Good Fats X

As much as possible, all foods organically grown, pasture-raised, and/ or purchased from local growers with minimum of packaging. X

Weaknesses: Need more variety in vegetable selections

Processed "foods"? ø

Grain-based foodstuffs? (Bread, bagels, chips, muffins, oatmeal, corn bread, cereals, sodas, cookies, crackers, grass-seed products) ø

High sugar dairy products? ø

Sugary liquids, sodas, and/or fruit juices)? Ø

Other: Black tea

2 oz. coconut manna/almond butter

Self-recommended Diet Changes: Purchase and prepare greater varieties of locally grown vegetables, herbs, and spices

*Note: Supplements taken each day: Fish oil; Vitamin D; Probiotic; Borage Oil

My Unique Recipes

I urge everyone to experiment with the recipes in ***Wheat Belly Total Health***, ***Grain Brain***, ***Gut and Psychology Syndrome***, ***Eat Fat Get Thin***, ***The Plant Paradox***, ***The Gut Balance Revolution***, and several of the other well-researched nutritional texts of the 21st Century. In the following pages, I present a few recipes of my own, which represent the efforts of someone who prefers to spend only very limited amounts of time preparing delicious and nutritious foods. Most of these "meals" can be transported easily to several different venues of activity during busy days.

Strength for Life® Trail Mix

2 ounces each	1 ounce each
1.Raw organic nuts	1.Raw Organic Sesame Seeds
1.Brazil	2.Dried mulberries
2.Almonds	D.1/4 teaspoon of organic spices
3.Pecans	1.cinnamon
4.Pistaschios	2.rosemary
B.Dried Organic Coconut flakes	3.turmeric
C.Raw organic seeds	4.ginger
1.Walnuts	5.oregano
	6. basil

Place all ingredients in a large Mason-type jar, fasten lid tightly; shake until mixed thoroughly. Shake periodically to prevent small seeds and spices from congregating at the bottom. Always purchase organic ingredients, locally grown whenever possible. All raw nuts and seeds should be refrigerated or stored in very cool and dry places and eaten within one month of purchase.

JA's Strongevity Protein Smoothie

This recipe is for approximately one quart. Often, I drink half for breakfast one day and the other half for breakfast the next day. Normally, I make this concoction at night, refrigerate it overnight in a Mason jar, and then transport it to work in a small cooler. On most days, I exercise for an hour first thing in the morning, having only water, a couple tablespoons of sauerkraut, and supplements beforehand. About half an hour after completing my training session, I begin sipping this smoothie as my breakfast/after-exercise meal. This powerhouse is packed with protein, fiber, beneficial fats, and other essential nutrients. If you do not have a blender, combine the ingredients in a large jar and shake vigorously for at least 30 seconds. However, you will enjoy this dynamo much more if it is blended thoroughly into a delicious, cold, thick froth.

Pour 12-16 ounces of water, coffee, or tea into a blender. Starting at a slow speed, through the opening in the cap, gradually add the following ingredients:

1. 2 ounces of Whey Protein powder from pasture-raised cows or goats, or Organic Hemp Protein powder;
2. 2 Tablespoons each of organic Flax seeds (ground), Sesame Seeds, and Fresh or Frozen Cranberries or Blueberries;
3. 1 Tablespoon each of Organic Walnuts, Pecans, or Almonds, Greens First Concentrated Vegetable Powder, Brewer's or Nutritional Yeast, and Organic Cacao or Maca Powder;
4. Two Tablespoons of Organic, Cold-pressed, Virgin Coconut Oil;
5. One teaspoon of Organic Cinnamon Powder.
6. Add 4-8 ounces of Organic Almond Protein Milk or more water. If you are drinking it immediately, add ice cubes. Increase the blender speed gradually to reach preferred consistency.
7. Pour into quart jar and refrigerate.

Salad in a Jar

This is another concoction I prepare at night, refrigerate overnight, and take to work the following morning in a small cooler with my protein smoothie.

In a large mixing bowl, I cut up my favorite greens into small to medium sized pieces. Then I add **1-2 ounces each of apple cider vinegar and olive oil**, followed by my favorite **spices, such as oregano, basil, turmeric, ginger, rosemary, garlic,** etc. I toss these around briefly to achieve a good mixture of ingredients. To this I then add whatever other vegetables, low-sugar fruits, and nuts I have on hand. Next, I add a few more teaspoons of vinegar and oil as needed and mix everything thoroughly. With a large spoon, I ladle the salad into a wide-mouth Mason jar, seal, and refrigerate. On most days at lunch, I eat the whole quart of salad. I usually accompany the salad with a leftover from the main course the night before or 3 to 4 soft-boiled eggs. If you are a vegan, try grilled tempeh.

Greens: I favor strong, slightly bitter greens, such as **dandelion greens, endive, mizuna, or beet greens**. If you prefer a more neutral green, **romaine lettuce** is excellent. Trying new greens as part of a salad in a jar is a great way to expand your vegetable repertoire. For more flavor and zip, add **sauerkraut and/or fermented red cabbage, scallions**, and, in season, **garlic scapes. Celery** always adds a great crunch to any salad.

Brightly colored vegetables and low-sugar fruits: I usually dice **carrots** and spoon **fermented beets** into my salads. They add color, character, and a little low-sugar sweetness to the ensemble. **Radishes, celery, green or red cabbage, olives, and slices of avocado** provide textural relief and a lot more flavor. Small **pieces of apple** seem to absorb the flavors and fluids from all the other characters in the cast and make the entire play more interesting.

Raw Nuts: Pistachios, walnuts, pecans, brazil nuts, almonds, and/or macadamia nuts add crunch, protein, and healthful fats to this mini-feast.

Other options: If you prefer a creamier dressing than just olive oil and apple cider vinegar, simply add a few tablespoons of lactose-free sour cream from pasture-raised cows or goats. A few dried mulberries add more sweetness and crunch.

48+ Hour Bone Broth

One of the most nutritious foods we can consume is bone broth, made simply by cooking animal bones, bone marrow, and connective tissues (ligaments, tendons, cartilage) in water on a low heat for an extended time, usually at least 48 hours. As a result of this slow-cooking process, the mineral constituents and proteins of these tough tissues are broken down into liquids and/or gelatins that are very readily absorbed in the digestive system of a human being who eats and drinks them. We can enjoy bone broth simply as a hot beverage by heating it in a sauce pan, stirring in a few preferred spices, and then drinking it in a mug. As such, it makes a great between-meal pick-me-up or a substitute for a caffeinated beverage. If we are adventurous enough to make our own soup at home, we can begin with bone broth as the base and simply add our favorite tasty vegetables.

Possibly the most wasteful characteristic of the current American diet occurs when we throw the bones of animals into the trash. If we were to make bone broth out of all the connective tissues of the animals we slaughter and consume in this nation, we would be much healthier and reduce drastically the number of animals we need to raise and slaughter. Quite simply, when we throw away the ingredients for bone broth, we are wasting vast amounts of valuable nutritional resources. Fortunately, all over the country, new breeds of butchers are opening old-time shops that offer meats only from pasture-raised animals. Many of these progressive purveyors of pure animal products not only sell the bones necessary to make your own bone broth at home, they also make 48+hour bone broth that we can simply take home and consume with almost no effort. However, for those who want to make their own bone broth, here are some directions.

From a pasture-raised butcher shop, purchase 2-4 pounds of animal bones with attached ligaments, tendons, cartilage, etc. Alternatively, purchase bone-in beef shanks or pork chops. Or save the carcass from a chicken or turkey. If there is still meat on the bones, cut off what you can, refrigerate it, and save it for later. In a large pot, place the bones et al on the bottom, then pour in pure water until the bones are submerged completely. Turn on medium heat and allow to cook but not quite boil. If you are using a large crock pot, you may simply allow the pot to cook at a low to medium heat for at least two days. If you are cooking on a stove top, you should turn the heat off at night and at any time when you are not at home. The broth will remain warm. When you are awake and/or return home, heat broth to a slight boil for a few minutes, then reduce to low heat. This method may require three days of cooking.

When the cooking period for the broth is nearly complete, turn off the heat and allow it to cool for a few hours. As it does, if you have any meat that you cut off the bones previously, sauté or bake it with a few vegetables. When the broth is cool, pour it through a strainer to separate any remaining solid matter. Compost the solid matter. Pour half of the broth into a Vitamix machine or a powerful blender. Add the cooked meat, veggies, clarified butter and your favorite spices. Blend the mixture thoroughly until the meat is gelatinous if not liquefied. Pour this mixture back into the remaining broth in the big pot, heat on a low flame, and stir until all is mixed thoroughly.

Once the broth is mixed, allow it to cool to room temperature, then pour it into one-quart containers, allowing at least two inches of open space at the top. Place the number of one-quart containers you will consume during the next seven days in the refrigerator. Whatever quantity of broth remains should be placed in the freezer or given to friends. Every omnivore should try to drink at least one glass of bone broth a day. On most days, I heat up a pint in a sauce pan in the morning and take it to work in a coffee mug. If I drink it as a mid-morning snack, it is still hot and luscious.

Making soup with a bone broth base could not be simpler. Simply put one quart of water and one quart of broth in a three-quart pan, turn on medium heat, and then add chopped up vegetables and spices. Allow to simmer—but not boil—for a fewhours until the vegetables are cooked but still firm.

Cabbasagna

Cabbasagna is merely traditional lasagna made with cabbage instead of lasagna noodles. From a nutritional point of view, we simply replace a fattening, addicting, and inflammatory, wheat-based foodstuff (lasagna noodles) with a highly nutritious vegetable (cabbage). In addition, we use strained tomatoes to eliminate the lectins in the seeds and skin of that fruit. Most other ingredients in traditional lasagna are healthful: ricotta or another cheese from pastured cows, organically grown vegetables and spices, and meat from pasture-raised animals if you want meat in your lasagna. The only other variable is whether to sauté the cabbage before baking or, if you like it crunchier, place it in the baking dish still raw.

JA's Cabbasagna

A. Ingredients
1. One pound of ground turkey: pasture-raised
2. One small head of organic purple cabbage
3. One large organic onion
4. Two large organic portabella mushrooms
5. Six stalks of organic celery
6. Three cloves of organic garlic
7. 16 ounces of strained tomatoes (drain excess water)
8. 8 ounces of cheddar cheese (from pasture-raised animals)
9. 8 ounces of sour cream (from pasture-raised animals)
10. Organic Pepper, salt, basil, oregano, ghee (clarified butter)

B. Procedure

1. On stove top with low heat in a stainless-steel pan, in order, add: 2 Tbsp. ghee; Turkey; Onion chopped; Garlic chopped; Celery, chopped; Mushrooms, chopped; ½ tsp. basil and oregano; ¼ tsp. pepper and salt. Cook 15 min.

2. Meanwhile, at 300 degrees in the oven in a large rectangular Pyrex glass dish, melt 1 Tbsp. ghee, then spread 1/3 of cabbage, chopped, over the bottom and allow to bake for 10 minutes.

3. When turkey and vegetables are lightly cooked, remove from stove top.

4. With large spoon, layer ½ of turkey/vegetables on top of cabbage.

5. Layer ½ of tomato, 1/3 of cabbage, then all sour cream; add spice to taste.

6. Layer the other half of the turkey/vegetables on top of sour cream.

7. Layer on the rest of the cabbage, then the rest of the tomato; return to oven to bake for 30 minutes

8. Grate cheese; remove Pyrex from oven; sprinkle on layer of cheese evenly; return to oven to bake 10-20 minutes.

To suit your personal tastes, you may choose to substitute other ingredients: pastured beef or pork for turkey; ricotta cheese instead of sour cream. I use purple instead of green cabbage because the result is a sweeter taste. The recipe above yields eight large servings.

Nutritional Supplements

Without question, nutritional supplements can be an important part of a healthy human diet. In many localities and/or because of seasonal climate changes, it may be almost impossible to get all the nutrients we need from available whole-food sources alone. In addition, many of us have individual health disorders that can be lessened or even cured with the addition of highly-concentrated nutrients found only in supplements. Therefore, all of us should consider supplements to augment the nutrients we absorb from the foods and beverages we eat and drink.

Because supplements are highly concentrated forms of nutrients, we must be as vigilant about the qualities of the ones we purchase as we are about the types and qualities of the foods we select. For one specific individual, high concentrations of certain nutrients in supplement form can be used to correct serious deficiencies or imbalances in his or her body. However, for another individual, the same dosage of the same supplement could be highly toxic or trigger an allergic reaction. For instance, ingesting self-prescribed doses of Vitamin A could be fatal for someone who really doesn't need this nutrient, especially in high amounts. Less dramatically, someone who ingests the wrong type of calcium or iron supplements may experience indigestion or constipation. In short, self-administered nutritional supplementation can be very risky. Therefore, it is essential that when considering nutritional supplements, we consult with a licensed healthcare provider who is well-educated and experienced in the fields of nutrition and supplementation.

There are at least four nutritional supplements which, I recommend, we should discuss with our health care providers: fish oil from certified pure sources to provide essential Omega-3 fatty acids that are difficult to obtain from foods; borage oil or evening primrose oil to provide an essential Omega-6 fatty acid that should be consumed in concert with fish oils; Vitamin D, a vitally important hormone which is difficult to get in sufficient quantities from food alone; and a probiotic to replenish the microorganisms we lose in great quantities every day.

Beyond those general guidelines, the use of nutritional supplements will not be covered in this book. We must remain focused on the big event. The primary purpose of *American Diet Revolution!* is to further the cause of a revolution in the whole foods we eat and in our understanding of these foods. Obviously, from a negative point of view, we must stop consuming the toxic, fattening, and nutritionally-deficient foods we have been deceived into eating since the 1950s. More importantly, from a positive perspective, we all must establish new, proactive dietary habits and resume consuming many of the foods that our ancestors ate with relish.

By expressing our freedom to choose foods that help us become lean and vibrant, we are revolting against those who exploited our gullibility in the past. The American Diet Revolution is not a diet plan; it is a war against enormously powerful economic enterprises that have no interest in seeing changes in the dietary habits of Americans. Over the last several decades, these Exploiters have established control at every available level of our society: in government, in industry, in academia, and in the media. As individuals, we cannot sit back and depend on some governmental agency or media entity to suddenly arise and lead the charge to reinstate truth, honesty, and good health as the primary motivations in the growing, distribution, and consumption of food in the United States. If we do not act individually—by rejecting and replacing colonizing foodstuffs and the forces behind them—we will continue to become more obese, more diabetic, and more disabled. If we do not first change radically the whole foods we eat, consuming concentrated supplements will not save our independence.

Chapter Eight

Economize, Ecologize, and Exercise: Armaments #3-5

On the personal battlefront in the American Diet Revolution, the two most powerful weapons each of us can utilize are: (1) Educating Ourselves and (2) Eating for Well-Being. Utilizing these armaments enables us to realize our individual potentials for health independence from the Exploiters, who profit most when we are uninformed, unquestioning, malnourished, obese, and prematurely disabled by preventable diseases—that is, patsies for colonization. Although the next two weapons—to Economize and "Ecologize"—can also benefit us personally, they are of even greater benefit to our fellow and sister citizens of local, national, and global communities. In this chapter, we'll look at effective ways each of us, as individuals, can use these weapons to wage civil war on the local, national, and planetary battlefronts.

To Economize

At first, when we think about economizing in our food purchases, we think of strategies to minimize our personal expenditures, ways to spend as little money as possible when we buy food.

In the short run, this may seem to be a wise tactic, but, in the fields of health, nutrition, and independence, it can be a highly counterproductive strategy. If we buy what seem to be inexpensive foods at a supermarket, we may feel as though we have saved money. However, if these cheap foods are low in nutritional value, packed in lead-lined cans, preserved with toxic additives, or high in the type of calories that cause us to gain excessive amounts of body fat, they are not a bargain at any level. Cheap foods—as well as foods we are tricked into believing are cheap—will eventually and inevitably lead to vastly higher medical expenses than we would have incurred if we had chosen to purchase healthier foods at slightly higher initial costs.

Buying seemingly cheap food is exactly how the Exploiters want us to behave. We think we are saving money when, in reality, we are making a reservation for a room in one of their premature disability centers. The takeaway is this: buying cheap food is not economizing. If, instead, we use our free-enterprise rights to make wise food purchases, we are employing a weapon that will not only save us money personally but will also benefit the human communities in which we live. The following is a list of several ways in which to wield this powerful economizing weapon.

1. Support your local community. As much as possible, buy organic foods:

    a. directly from local organic growers at farmers' markets, on-premise farm stands, through farm shares, etc.;

    b. at local food co-ops, which always specialize in locally grown foods and whose staff members are dedicated to high principles in food production and distribution;

c. at local health food stores that feature locally-grown, organic produce;

d. at local supermarkets that carry local organic foods;

e. at local butcher shops carrying pasture-raised animal products exclusively.

Every food dollar we spend locally reverberates throughout our local communities. It is especially important that we honor our local organic growers by purchasing the foods they work so hard to produce. We may pay a little more for the extra physical labor that small-scale farming requires, but the nutritional health benefits from eating exquisitely fresh organic produce and pastured animal products repay us tenfold throughout the course of our lifetimes.

2. Purchase as little processed food as possible. The more processing a food undergoes before you purchase it, the greater the percentage of your money that goes toward such processing. Each middleman along the processed food chain sucks out his profits. You pay for his processing, his additives, his packaging, his handling, his transportation costs, etc. The more you pay middlemen, the less nutrition you receive for your food dollar investments. A few examples follow.

a. Instead of buying a box of breakfast cereal that has been shipped across the country, make your own delicious breakfast crunchola by purchasing raw seeds, nuts, and spices in bulk from your local food co-op or health food store and adding some local organic blueberries.

b. Instead of buying a box of frozen chicken parts from some industrial chicken factory or buying a feedlot steak sitting on foam and wrapped in plastic at a six-acre supermarket, go to your local butcher who sells only fresh, local, pasture-raised meats and ask him or her to provide you with a cut of exactly what you want. Without question, you will find the local, pasture-raised meat to be more flavorful than the injected facsimiles sold under mesmerizing lights at a super-duper market. You will also discover that you are satisfied with a much smaller serving of the local meat than you are with a larger hunk of its industrial counterpart. You will be economizing personally by eating less of a high-quality nutritious and delicious food than you would have eaten if you had consumed a much larger portion of a toxic, overly-processed, antibiotic-laden meatstuff. In addition, you will be economizing on the local, national, and global battlefronts as well. You will be supporting your neighboring business person. You will be reducing unnecessary national transportation, packaging, and chemical disposal costs, which will lessen the carbon impact of your food choices on the air, land, and seas. The environmental impact of individual choices may seem small. However, when multiplied by hundreds of millions of people, the beneficial economic and environmental effects are profound.

3. One of the least economizing ways to use our food dollars is to patronize fat-fast-food "restaurants." Foodstuffs at these highway carnival sideshows are extremely processed, adulterated with excessive amounts of cheap sugars, salts, and other additives, and wrapped in grain-based doughs and vast amounts of throwaway plastics, papers, and other pollutants. Withdrawing our financial support—by depatronizing these emporiums of obesity and illness—is one of the most effective weapons we can use in our revolution against colonization by obesity and disease.

4. One other economic weapon of revolt against our colonization by obesity is to cease ordering crusted wheat slabs known as

pizzas from national chains and other bakeries that still use wheat to make their pizza crusts and other baked "goods." By now, we should all know that wheat-based foodstuffs are bait used to addict and fatten human beings. The nutritional value of a grain-based pizza crust is miniscule, outweighed by the toxicity of those grains to the human GI tract and their ability to rapidly raise our blood sugar levels, thereby triggering an insulin reaction and the cascade of illness events that follow that reaction. There are now growing numbers of bakers in localities throughout the country who use seed- and nut-based flours to make baked products. In the recipes in **Wheat Belly Total Health**, William Davis gives instructions for making pizza with a flax-seed crust. We economize when we patronize grain-free bakeries or try grain-free baking recipes at home.

To Ecologize

Buying and eating organic, pasture-raised, and locally grown foods are potent socioeconomic weapons. In wielding these armaments, we are supporting an offensive by the American Diet Revolutionary Army to slow down destruction of the habitability of planet Earth for human beings.

a. Consume locally raised foods to minimize the transportation pollution caused by the incineration of fossil fuels during transcontinental and international shipping.

b. Purchase foods with as little packaging as possible to preserve trees, oil, water, soil, and virtually every other natural resource.

c. Read food labels carefully. Buy foods identified as being "GMO-free", "Fair-Trade", and organically grown.

If we extend the philosophy of purchasing the purest possible foods to the other financial purchases we make—cleaners, shampoos, toothpaste, household and business items, auto, house, and yard maintenance—we put economic pressure on manufacturers of all sizes and locations to make more planet-friendly products to meet our demands. Once again, thoughtful purchases are potent weapons of liberation. If we practice internal environmentalism and external environmentalism simultaneously, we can free ourselves from the clutches of those who thrive by exploiting us.

All of us, both individually and collectively, must consider the implications of unlimited growth in the human population upon the global battlefront. Indeed, it is possible—actually probable—we have exceeded already the number of human beings who can live on our planet in peace, harmony, and excellent health and who can enjoy the blessings and beauty of Nature. This idea runs counter to the goals of titanic enterprises, symbolized by groups such as the Exploiters, that thrive on continuing expansion in the populations of potential customer profit centers. These titans want to delay any substantive discussion of soaring CO_2 concentrations, increasing global temperatures, melting glaciers, rising sea levels, expanding "dead zones" in oceans and lakes, etc. Rather than envisioning a world in which the population of human beings gradually declines, so that we can live within the capacity of our planet to sustain us, they prefer to picture skyscrapers built on arching steel foundations spanning the Grand Canyon. Just think of how many potential new consumers they could service if the entire North American continent were covered with vertical housing structures!

A few well-meaning philanthropists have helped fund efforts to increase the production of grains throughout the world, especially in nations with large populations of people living at the edge of starvation. They have been told that the only way to feed so many people is with grain-based foodstuffs. They realize that our planet cannot possibly offer to all human beings the types and quantities of the foods that they—and the rest of us in the "developed world"—enjoy. Therefore, they pour billions of dollars into the worldwide expansion of grain production to feed the masses. Their goals are noble; their hearts and souls are devoted to concern for their fellow and sister citizens of the Earth. But, given the knowledge we now have about the ill-health effects of predominantly grain-based diets, these charitable efforts are funding a vast expansion of human disease. **Grains are the fossil fuels of the human diet**. We can eat them and use their calories for the energy to carry on with our lives. However, they are the equivalent of burning coal in our houses to stay warm in winter and cook food year-round. Just as the byproducts of burning coal accumulate in our air, water, and land, so the byproducts of burning modern grains in our bodies accumulate in our tissues. These byproducts are known as Advanced Glycation Endproducts (AGEs). They congregate in every organ system. The human body cannot eliminate these pollutants. Our health is seriously compromised by these accumulating substances. This is great news for the Exploiters because they can profit immensely by keeping us alive in a dependent state for many years—taking their expensive medications, requiring intensive 24-hour care in their institutions, and still eating their mushy, grain-based foodstuffs.

To many, the last two paragraphs may seem to be a cynical caricature of the Big Three Enterprises of Health: Big Farma, Big Pharma, and the Medical Industrial Complex. But the sad reality is that they want us to continue eating as we have since the 1950s and marching into their institutions of colonization. However, each of us has the capability to fight back, to liberate ourselves from their greedy clutches, and to help our friends, neighbors, and loved ones break free as well. The first step toward liberation is to eat in a manner we now know is beneficial to our personal health. The second step is to help our loved ones and neighbors educate themselves and apply their knowledge to what they eat and what they think about what they eat. The third step is to speak or write to well-intentioned philanthropists, who feel as though they are doing the right thing but are actually reinforcing the status quo.

It is the responsibility of every citizen on planet Earth, to the greatest extent of which each of us is capable, to conserve our natural resources. As American Diet Revolutionaries, we must endeavor to make our food (and other) purchases with as little packaging as possible, especially plastic and other non-biodegradable packaging. In addition, we must recycle every bit of packaging we do use, as well as all other reusable materials ready for disposal. Our oceans are now so polluted with plastic waste that finding even wild-caught fish without plastic residuals in their tissues has become extremely difficult. To recycle is to revolt against the could-care-less economic giants who profit most when we are not careful.

To Exercise:

If and how we exercise has a profound impact on how well we eat. How well we eat has a profound impact on how well we exercise. Exercising with excellence but eating poorly leads to relatively poor health. It is better than if you did not exercise at all, but far inferior to how healthy you could be, if you were eating for well-being. Eating well but exercising poorly, or not at all, leads to substandard health. Again, it is better than if you ate poorly, but vastly inferior to how healthy you could be, if you were exercising as well as you were eating.

In short, exercise is an essential element of a truly healthy diet and vice versa.

Exercise influences our diet in several ways. First, exercising vigorously stimulates our sense of thirst, causing us to drink more fluids than if we were sedentary. If we are "on the ball," most of the fluid we drink is pure water rather than some expensive, psychedelically-colored, pseudo-health, sports drink. Drinking ample amounts of unadulterated water facilitates efficient elimination of waste products.

Secondly, exercising influences when we eat. If we are thoughtful about our exercise habits, most of us abstain from eating solid food for at least one hour prior to beginning a vigorous bout of exertion. During an intensive workout and for a brief period afterward, the desire to eat solid food is suppressed. However, approximately half an hour later, our sense of hunger is heightened, causing us to eat more food than if we had been sitting at a computer for the previous few hours.

Thus, exercise affects not only the times at which we eat, but also the quantities of food we eat. Research shows that when we exercise regularly, we consume more calories than when we are inactive. This is one reason why exercise alone, without the benefit of eating intelligently, is not an effective approach to reducing body fat.

Exercise also affects our diet by influencing the types and qualities of food we eat. For example, if you do abdominal exercises daily (as we all should) you will not be inclined to bloat your belly with large bowls of pasta or cereal or with big slices of pizza. If you do make this mistake, you will experience the very unpleasant sensation of feeling your abdomen stretch forward, outward, and downward against the resistance of muscles you have been training to pull backward, inward, and upward. Psychologically, eating this poorly after exercising intelligently is equivalent to washing and waxing your car and then immediately driving it out into a muddy cornfield to practice wheelies and spinouts.

Physiologically, exercise has pronounced effects upon digestion. Vigorous contractions of skeletal muscles, especially during whole-body forms of exertion, such as running, jumping, or dancing, stimulate haustrations, the smooth muscle contractions that move food and waste products through the human GI tract. On the other hand, gentler forms of physical exertion, such as the rhythmic movements of a low-intensity stroll shortly after a meal, also stimulate haustrations, as well as keep your blood sugar level lower than if you had chosen instead to sit in front of a computer or television.

Considered from the opposite point of view, what and how we eat influences how—and even if—we exercise. When we eat foods containing indigestible lectin proteins, as found in most grain-based foodstuffs and legumes, we experience gastric distress that may last for hours and prevent us from even considering a vigorous bout of exercise for one, two, or even three days. When we eat foods that raise our blood sugar levels rapidly, such as sugary and/or grainy foodstuffs, we trigger an insulin reaction that often lowers our blood sugar levels to the point where we feel tired, sluggish, and more inclined to nap than to exercise.

What we eat also impacts our exercise habits in subtle ways. If we eat large amounts of foods high in pro-inflammatory, Omega-6 fatty acids, such as grain-based foodstuffs or animal products derived from creatures raised on grains, we are likely to experience joint and muscle pains. We may not be aware of its cause, but the musculoskeletal pain will definitely discourage us from exercising.

Another way what we eat influences how or if we exercise is by supplying or not supplying essential nutrients after a vigorous exercise session. If we eat nutritious foods between our bouts of exercise, our bodies assimilate the nutrients from these foods and use them to rebuild the muscle tissue broken down during each exercise session. We feel our strength and energy levels increasing.

By contrast, if our diets do not furnish us with the healthy supply of high-quality protein and digestive cofactors we need, we do not rebuild muscle tissue, do not grow stronger, and have increased pain in our weakly muscled joints.

Stated simply: a poor diet discourages us from exercising; an excellent diet increases the benefits of our exercise efforts.

To become a healthy American Diet Revolutionary, there are several dimensions of fitness we can strive for by exercising intelligently. Below is a list of eight dimensions of potential health improvement.

1. Increased Strength
2. Increased Muscle and Bone Mass
3. Increased Flexibility
4. Improved Cardiorespiratory Fitness
5. Improved Posture
6. Improved Balance, Equilibrium, Agility, Coordination
7. Improved Digestion
8. Decreased Body Fat

If we integrate a comprehensive exercise program with a highly conscientious approach to eating for well-being, we are capable of reaching higher states of health and fitness than we could attain by practicing only one of these vital disciplines.

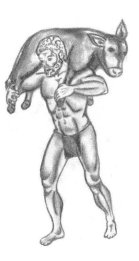

Milo of Croton was a five-time Gold Medalist at the pan-Grecian Olympic Games. He developed his supreme level of whole-body fitness by running through fields and woods with a calf draped over his shoulders. His diet was the real Mediterranean Diet and a forerunner of the American Revolutionary Diet.

Chapter Nine

Recapitulation: Let's Face the Music and Take Back Our Health Freedom

The types of foods we eat today—and have been eating in great quantities since the 1950s—are, by far, the major reason why so many of us have gained large amounts of unwanted body fat and/or become diabetic during this era. Without question, we accepted dietary advice from paid-off researchers, governmental agencies, medical groups, and industrial organizations we assumed were primarily motivated to help us become leaner and healthier and enable us "to enjoy life, liberty, and the pursuit of happiness."

Our trust was misplaced.

We know now that before we trust our health to others, we must learn to trust ourselves. We cannot rely on an individual, group, industry, or agency to take care of us. Each of us must be our own primary health provider.

In the last half of the 20th Century, many of the individuals and organizations that pretended to offer scientific dietary advice to the public were really promoting their own self-interests.

They exploited us.

As several independent researchers of the 21st Century have documented, the financial success for many of these individuals and groups was and is directly related to the percentages of us who are obese, diabetic, and/or otherwise disabled by eating foods that cause us to become their dependents, their sickly colonists.

If we peer into the future, these Exploiters have absolutely no financial incentive to see more of us become leaner and healthier. They thrive on the status quo. They continue to spew their propaganda to keep us colonized, addicted to the foods and drugs from which they profit profusely. Unfortunately, even today, most of us continue to follow their 20th Century dietary advice. We haven't been able to change our eating habits, in most cases because we have been relentlessly bombarded with their dietary deceptions for such a long period of time that we simply cannot let go of that bad advice.

Therefore, rather than continuing to trust the Exploiters to feed us all we know about nutrition, we must educate ourselves. Instead of swallowing TV food and drug ads hook, line, sinker, and pole, we must read books and articles about which foods are beneficial to our well-being and which food imposters are toxic to our bodily systems. Instead of permitting internet ad bait to be our primary source of dietary learning, we must navigate to sites where we can read clinical nutritional studies in their entirety. We cannot continue to accept unsubstantiated dietary advice as we did throughout the last half of the 20th Century.

The time is now to face the music. No longer can we be silent, accepting colonists. We have the capacity to liberate ourselves from oppression by misinformation and reclaim our right to health freedom. The real nutritional researchers of the 21st Century have given us the democratic armaments to do this, to revolt against those who have taken advantage of our trust, our good will, and our passive acceptance of information we should have studied and questioned thoughtfully in the past.

If we listen carefully, in the distance, we can hear a fife and drum corps beginning to march.

Our first volley of fire in the revolt against colonization by obesity, diabetes, and other diet-induced diseases is to shoot down the most damaging dietary advice myth of the 20th Century: that we should eat large quantities of "whole healthy grains."

How can we question the truth of this phrase?

Were we not advised by the United States Department of Agriculture in their Great Holy Food Pyramid of 1992 to eat seven to 11 servings of whole grain foods every day?

If ever there were a dietary recommendation to gain fat weight, this was it—and is still today. More than 50 percent of the calories we consume come from highly-processed, technologically-modified, grain-based foodstuffs—modern variants of wheat, corn, rice, and oats. If we are considering dietary causes of obesity, does it not seem logical that we should consider first the foods from which we ingest the most calories? However, we have been bludgeoned for decades with the unsubstantiated statement, "Eating grains is good for us." Therefore, we dismiss, without careful consideration, any claim that the genetically altered grains of today are detrimental to our health. Many of us have been trying to lose unwanted body fat for years. Despite evidence to the contrary, in the back of our minds, we tell ourselves:

"It can't be the grains, they are good for us."

"Look how many bakeries there are, and how big the bread and cereal aisles are in the supermarkets. It couldn't be possible that all that food is bad for us."

"Most of the foods I eat come from grains. I could not possibly survive if I stopped eating them entirely."

It is time for all of us to take our little fingers away from our closed eyelids and remove our thumbs from our ear canals.

The whistles of the fifes and the beats of the drums are even louder now. Members of the marching corps are stomping over the bloated carcass of the tired old "healthy-whole-grain" myth. **Grains are the fossil fuels of the human diet**. If we consume them, our bodies can use them for fuel, just as we can power our homes by burning coal and wood in open pits in our basements. However, smoke and creosote from the consumption and gastrointestinal combustion of grain-based foodstuffs have been choking us for decades. The time is now, at last, to release our minds and our bodies from the haze of the "healthy-whole-grain" myth. Through the thick smog of deceit, the music of a 21st Century revolutionary band has come to lead us away from the dirty dietary myths of the 20th Century.

Admitting that many of the foods which have dominated our diets since the 1950s are toxic is only the first crucial step toward reclaiming our health freedom. Our next essential rebellious act must be to replace those pathogenic foodstuffs in our old diets with new foods that supply our bodies with the nutrients we need to perform all the tasks of our daily lives with excellence. Therefore, our new diets will include many traditional foods (such as eggs or butter) which our ancestors ate, but we were urged to avoid during the Big Grain/Big Sugar/Low-fat Era. Our new revolutionary diets will also include several foods that many of us have never attempted to consume before, such as bone broth, mizuna, or dandelion greens.

During the 21st Century, several outstanding writer/physicians (Davis, Perlmutter, Campbell-McBride, Gedgaudas, Mullin, Gundry) have published extensive menus and delicious recipes based on the principles of what real, contemporary, nutritional research reveals to be foods healthful for human beings. By following their detailed dietary plans, we can supply our bodies with the nutrients we need to reach our individual potentials for health excellence and freedom. In *American Diet Revolution!* I attempt only to supplement, rather than duplicate, their superb efforts. Although earlier I presented a few of my own unique recipes and dietary recommendations, my primary intention is to consolidate and summarize the essential nutritional recommendations of these earlier authors. Therefore, in the following pages, I offer a concise, convenient, informational tool we can refer to quickly and easily as we make food decisions.

"The Two-Page, Pro-Active, Strength for Life®**Every-Single-Day, Eating-for-Well-Being Guide,"** is a succinct instrument to remind ourselves which foods and beverages we should eat and drink and which foods we should avoid. However, as we implement these guidelines, we must remind ourselves to be patient. This is an ideal diet. We do not have to implement every dietary recommendation instantaneously or perfectly. On the first day, we do not have to eat and drink every food and beverage in the first section, the Essentials. Likewise, most of us will not be able to able to avoid immediately every toxic foodstuff in the third section, the Toxins. It is my recommendation, therefore, that we make dietary changes gradually. In the first week, each of us should choose one food from "the Essentials" section that we have not been eating and try adding it to our diets. During the next week, we should select one industrial foodstuff from "the Toxins" section and eliminate that type of food. If we introduce new foods into our diets in this manner, our gastrointestinal systems will have ample time to adjust. Plus, removing incrementally the toxic foods that disrupt the GI tract will facilitate a smooth transition to a calmer and more pleasing state of digestive health. Over a period of a few months, each of us will develop a personal repertoire of foods that facilitate a high level of personal health. Then, when we look back at our weekly food diaries during this period, we will be amazed at how quickly and efficiently we replaced the intestinal chaos and disease cacophony caused by 20th Century dietary advice with personal, 21st Century, nutritional harmony and health.

The Two-Page, Pro-Active, Strength for Life®, Every-Single-Day, Eating-for-Well-Being Guide

What <u>We</u> <u>Must</u> <u>Eat</u> <u>and</u> <u>Drink</u>: the Essentials

1. **Eat 7-10 servings of fresh, local, organic vegetables, including:**
   a. a large salad with raw, leafy greens and brightly colored vegetables;
   b. at least one full cup of lightly cooked vegetables and/or soup;
   c. at least two ounces of fermented vegetables, such as sauerkraut.
2. **Eat several servings of local, organic and/or pastured-raised fats, including:**
   a. at least two tablespoons of coconut oil, olive oil, and/or ghee; and
   b. at least 2-4 ounces of raw nuts, olives, and/or avocado; and/or
   c. 2-3 ounces of animal fat in eggs, ghee, meat, or fish (ova/omnivores).
3. **Eat 2-4 ounces of organic/pasture-raised proteins at 2-3 meals, such as:**
   a. 2-3 eggs, if you are an ova-lactivore or omnivore; and/or
   b. 2 ounces of raw nuts; and/or
   c. 2-4 ounces of bone, meat, or fish protein, if you are an omnivore.
4. **Drink at least three pints of pure water—one pint between all meals.**
5. **Drink at least two servings of nutritional beverages, such as:**
   a. 1-2 cups of bone broth, if you are an omnivore; and/or
   b. 1-2 cups of a high-mineral vegetable broth or drink; and/or
   c. 8-16 ounces of a nutritional smoothie, especially post-exercise;
   d. home-made, vegetable-rich, and/or bone-broth-based soups.

What <u>We</u> <u>May</u> <u>Eat</u> <u>or</u> <u>Drink</u>: the Optionals

1. 1-2 servings of organic low-sugar fruit, especially red, purple, blue berries;
2. 1-2 cups of coffee, tea, or kombucha, and 3-6 ounces of organic red wine;
3. 1-4 ounces of pasture-raised butter, cheese, sour cream, whole-milk yogurt;
4. 1-2 ounces of an organic chocolate bar, ≥ 80 percent cacao, ≤ 3 grams of sugar;
5. 2-3 ounces of organic cooked fermented soy, or baked sweet potato;
6. and, once per week, a "goof" (e.g., ice cream at your favorite parlor).

What <u>We</u> <u>Must</u> <u>Eliminate</u>: the Toxins

1. All processed, non-organic, genetically modified, or artificially sweetened, flavored, colored, or preserved foods, including but not limited to:
   a. industrial foodstuffs derived from plants treated with herbicides, pesticides, fungicides, or chemical fertilizers;
   b. foods from animals treated with antibiotics or growth stimulants or fed chemically-raised grains or other toxins.
2. All grain-based foodstuffs, including: breads, pasta, cereals, oatmeal, bagels, granola, crackers, cookies, pizza, muffins, scones, pies, cakes.
3. All sugar-intense or artificially sweetened: beverages (fruit juices, sodas, sweetened teas, coffees, or sports drinks); solid foods (candies, cookies, pastries, low-fat and non-fat dairy products, or foodstuffs sweetened with high-fructose corn syrup and facsimiles).

4. All high-lectin and/or starchy pseudo-vegetable foods, such as: tomatoes, nightshades, beans, peanuts, corn, potatoes, fries, popcorn, chips, etc.

5. All foods containing inflammatory, high Omega-6, pseudo-vegetable oils, such as: corn, soybean, cottonseed, canola, safflower, peanut, sunflower.

6. As much as possible, any foods or drinks that cause GI distress, such as gas or bloating, or are sold in metal cans, plastic bags, or plastic containers.

Coda

To Arms! To Arms!

They came, they saw, and they conquered us—temporarily.

The Exploiters capitalized on an opportunity to dominate a passively acceptant citizenry in a free-enterprise socioeconomic system. Stealthily, they built empires by seizing control of what we eat and what we think about what we eat. By infiltrating the organizations that advise us about what we should eat, they seduced us into buying and eating food commodities from which they profit most and over which they have the most control. As a result, unparalleled numbers of American citizens are obese, pathologically overweight, diabetic, neurologically impaired, and otherwise physically and mentally compromised. We are their de facto colonists.

As all empires built on self-proclaimed righteousness and greed, that of the Exploiters will fall. Their descent will result not primarily from their own excessive pride and thirst for power, but rather, from a spirited uprising among their subjects, namely, from us.

When American colonists first declared their rights to independence from England, very few believed they would succeed in their quest. Rag-tag rebels versus a great military power? No way! But, yes! Indeed!

The American Diet Revolution is an opportunity to correct a terrible wrong—the passive surrender of our health freedom to vested interest groups, agricultural and chemical corporations, political agencies, medical organizations, and other industries that profit most when a majority of us are disabled by obesity and related diet-induced diseases. Fortunately for us, the rebels who created the first national democracy gave us the rights and responsibilities to improve and maintain that democracy. But we must exercise those rights and responsibilities.

Today, one of the most essential of those responsibilities is to educate ourselves about food, to refuse to accept dogma or dog food from anyone, especially from master brewers of foods and information that make us fat and drugs that make us addicted dependents. Actively educating ourselves about which foods help us become leaner and healthier is the ammunition for our liberation.

Another responsibility we must exercise is to shoulder the armaments of our newly gained nutritional knowledge. Purchasing and eating foods we know are healthy for us is a powerful socioeconomic weapon. Eating for well-being is to volunteer for active duty. In doing so, we are engaging in the fight for health freedom against vast and vague financial pharaohs of national and international commerce.

We Americans have the strength, the character, and the heritage to revolt against those who would like to keep us colonized, those who stand to lose substantial amounts of money and power when we exercise our right to strive for well-being. May *American Diet Revolution!* inspire you to exercise your right to participate personally and actively in this revolution.

To arms! To arms!

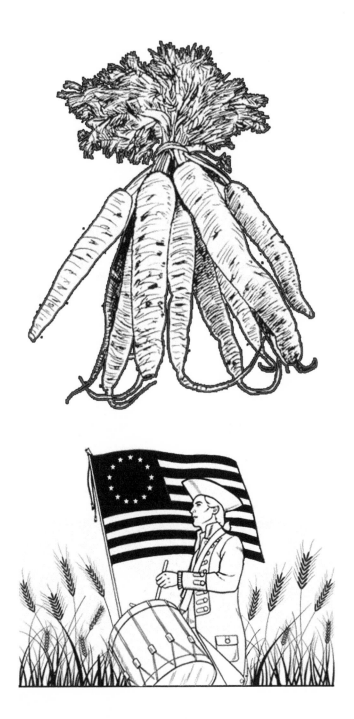

Thank you!

Thank you, dear reader, for taking the time to read ***American Diet Revolution!*** I hope you will become personally involved by joining an international online community of other thoughtful people devoted to learning and doing all they can about their own health, about the health of our fellow citizens, and about the health of our planet. If you visit StrengthForLife.com, you will discover an exciting and continually expanding series of learning tools for the 21st Century. Our offerings include not only information about diet and nutrition, but also about ways to exercise safely and effectively, environmentalism, mental and spiritual health, and much more. You will have direct access to timely blogposts, podcasts, webinars, videocasts, newsletters, and eBooks. These instruments of modern communication will help you keep up-to-date with many important developments about health and well-being in our constantly challenging contemporary world. As a token of thanks, please opt in to our free online learning center at StrengthforLife.com and download two complimentary bonuses:

1. **The Strength for Life® One-week Nutritional Diary**—a very convenient form to help you make superbly healthy food choices; and

2. ***Revolutionary Recipes for a Healthy American Diet***—an exciting new ebook with dozens of recipes, menus, cooking techniques, and innovative baking tips to help you put into

practice the nutritional principles of *__American Diet Revolution!__* This work was created as a group effort by members of the Strength for Life® community. You will find this book to be a very useful and practical way to expand your personal repertoire of delicious and nutritious foods.

About the Author

Even in his early childhood, Josef Arnould enjoyed the quest for physical fitness. Whether it was catching snakes, climbing trees, throwing rocks and snowballs, or hitting baseballs, he loved the thrill of physical exertion. As a voracious teenage reader, he was also stimulated by the relationship of good nutrition to successful athletic performance.

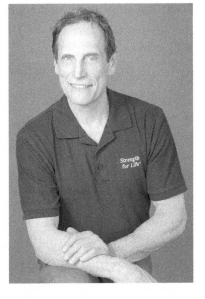

After graduating from Princeton University and Framingham State University, with bachelor's and master's degrees in English and Language Arts respectively, he entered Palmer College of Chiropractic with a career ambition of helping others achieve good health. In the curriculum at Palmer, he studied human anatomy, physiology, and nutrition in great depth.

Upon receiving his doctorate in 1983, Dr. Arnould opened a clinic in Western Massachusetts. From his first days of practice, he was determined to fuse three natural disciplines of health: whole-body exercise; nutritious eating; and comprehensive chiropractic healthcare. To symbolize his commitment to this concept, he named his practice

Strength for Life® Health and Fitness Center. Now in its 35th year, this clinic thrives as a community where people of all ages come to learn about exercising and eating intelligently and about receiving chiropractic care when necessary.

To share the knowledge and experience he had gained from many years of reading and teaching, as well as his lifelong love of exercise, Dr. Arnould composed a comprehensive textbook, *Stronger After 40: Strength Training as Healthcare for Women and Men in the 21st Century.* Published by Alward Publications in 2005, this work contains hundreds of photos and detailed explanations demonstrating how we can perform strength training and flexibility exercises safely and well, even if we are 80 or 90 years of age.

Now in his seventies, Dr. Arnould keeps us up-to-date in the exploding field of nutrition, with an exciting new book, *American Diet Revolution!* Much more than a manual of dietary advice, in this work we learn why and how, if we value our own health and the health of everyone we know and love, we must become activists about the foods we purchase and eat. Instead of an appeal for your relaxed consideration, this book challenges you to take action!

Josef Arnould, D.C.
Author of *Stronger After 40* and *Abdominal Strength for Life*
Director of Strength for Life® Health & Fitness Center
Easthampton, Massachusetts
StrengthForLife.com

References

Anderson, Keaven, William Castelli, Daniel Levy, "Cholesterol Mortality: 30 Years of Follow-up from the Framingham Study." *Journal of the American Medical Association* **257**, no.16 (April 24,1987): 2176-2187. doi:10.1001/jama.1987.0339060062027

Campbell-McBride, Natasha. *Gut and Psychology Syndrome: Natural Treatment for Autism, Dyspraxia, A.D.D., Dyslexia, A.D.H.D., Depression, and Schizophrenia.* **Wymondham, Norfolk, United Kingdom: Medinform Publishing, Revised edition, 2010.**

Put Your Heart in Your Mouth: Natural Treatment for Atherosclerosis, Angina, Heart Attack, High Blood Pressure, Stroke, Arrhythmia, and Peripheral Vascular Disease. **Wymondham, Norfolk, United Kingdom: Medinform Publishing, Revised edition, 2016.**

Centers for Disease Control and Prevention. "Trends in Intake of Energy and Macronutrients in the United States 1971-2000." Morbidity and Mortality Weekly Report 53, no. 4 (February 6, 2004): 80-82.

Davis, William. *Wheat Belly.* New York: Rodale, 2011.

Wheat Belly Total Health: The Ultimate Grain-Free Health and Weight-Loss Life Plan. **New York: Rodale, 2014.**

Gedgaudas, Nora. *Primal Fat Burner: Live Longer, Slow Aging, Super-Power Your Brain and Save Your Life with a High-Fat, Low-Carb Paleo Diet.* **New York: Atria Books, 2017.**

Gundry, Steven. *The Plant Paradox: The Hidden Dangers in "Healthy" Foods That Cause Disease and Weight Gain.* New York: Harper Wave, 2017.

Howard, Barbara, Linda Van Horn, Judith Hisa, et al. "Low-Fat Dietary Pattern and Risk of Cardiovascular Disease: The Women's Health Initiative Randomized Controlled Dietary Modification Trial." Journal of the American Medical Association 295, no. 6 (February 8, 2006) 655-666. doi:10.1001/jama.2017.16974

Howard, Barbara, JoAnn Manson, Marcia Stefanick, et al. "Low-Fat Dietary Pattern and Weight Change Over 7 Years: The Women's Health Initiative Randomized Controlled Dietary Modification Trial." Journal of the American Medical Association 295, no. 1 (January 4, 2006): 39-49. doi:10.1001/jama.295.1.39

Hyman, Mark. *Eat Fat, Get Thin: Why the Fat We Eat is the Key to Sustained Weight Loss and Vibrant Health.* New York: Little, Brown and Company, 2016.

Krause, Ronald and Darlene Dreon. "Low-density-lipoprotein Subclasses and Response to a Low-fat Diet in Healthy Men." American Journal of Clinical Nutrition 62, no. 2, supplement (August 1995): 478-487s.

Masley, Stephen and Jonny Bowdon. *Smart Fat: Eat More Fat, Lose More Weight, Get Healthy Now.* New York: Harper One, 2017.

Mullin, Gerard. *The Gut Balance Revolution: Boost Your Metabolism, Restore Your Inner Ecology, and Lose the Weight for Good.* New York: Rodale, 2015.

Perlmutter, David. *Brain Maker: The Power of Gut Microbes to Heal and Protect Your Brain for Life.* New York: Little, Brown and Company, 2015.

Grain Brain: The Surprising Truth About Wheat, Carbs, and Sugar—Your Brain's Silent Killers. New York: Little, Brown and Company, 2013.

Prentice, Ross, Bette Caan, Rowan Chlebowski, et al. "Low-fat Dietary Pattern and Risk of Invasive Breast Cancer: The Women's Health Initiative Randomized Controlled Dietary Modification Trial." Journal of the American Medical Association 295, no.6 (February 8, 2006): 629-642. doi:10.1001/jama.295.6.629.

Ravnskov, Uffe. *The Cholesterol Myth: Exposing the Fallacy that Saturated Fats and Cholesterol Cause Heart Disease.* Washington, D.C.: New Trends, 2000.

Taubes, Gary. *The Case Against Sugar.* New York: Anchor Books, 2017. *Good Calories, Bad Calories: Challenging the Conventional Wisdom on Diet, Weight Control, and Disease.* New York: Alfred A. Knopf, 2007.

Why We Get Fat: And What to Do About It. New York: Anchor Books, 2011.

Teicholz, Nina. *The Big Fat Surprise: Why Butter, Meat and Cheese Belong in a Healthy Diet.* New York: Simon & Schuster, 2014.